101 Medication Tips for People with Diabetes

Betsy A. Carlisle, PharmD
Lisa A. Kroon, PharmD
Mary Anne Koda-Kimble, PharmD, CDE

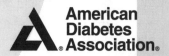

American Diabetes Association

Book Acquisitions	Robert J. Anthony
Editor	Laurie Guffey
Production Director	Carolyn R. Segree
Production Coordinator	Peggy M. Rote
Composition	Harlowe Typography, Inc.
Cover Design	Wickham & Associates, Inc.
Printer	Transcontinental Printing, Inc.

Printed in Canada
1 3 5 7 9 10 8 6 4 2

The suggestions and information contained in this publication are generally consistent with the *Clinical Practice Recommendations* and other policies of the American Diabetes Association, but they do not represent the policy or position of the Association or any of its boards or committees. Reasonable steps have been taken to ensure the accuracy of the information presented. However, the American Diabetes Association cannot ensure the safety or efficacy of any product or service described in this publication. Individuals are advised to consult a physician or other appropriate health care professional before undertaking any diet or exercise program or taking any medication referred to in this publication. Professionals must use and apply their own professional judgment, experience, and training and should not rely solely on the information contained in this publication before prescribing any diet, exercise, or medication. The American Diabetes Association—its officers, directors, employees, volunteers, and members—assumes no responsibility or liability for personal or other injury, loss, or damage that may result from the suggestions or information in this publication.

ADA titles may be purchased for business or promotional use or for special sales. For information, please write to Lee M. Romano, Special Sales & Promotions, at the address below.

American Diabetes Association
1660 Duke Street
Alexandria, Virginia 22314

Library of Congress Cataloging-in-Publication Data

Carlisle, Betsy A., 1960–
    101 medication tips for people with diabetes / Betsy A. Carlisle,
Lisa A. Kroon, Mary Anne Koda-Kimble.
      p.   cm.
    Includes bibliographical references and index.
    ISBN 1-58040-032-9 (pbk.)
    1. Diabetes—Chemotherapy Miscellanea. 2. Hypoglycemic agents
Miscellanea. I. Kroon, Lisa A., 1970– . II. Koda-Kimble, Mary
Anne. III. Title. IV. Title: One hundred one medication tips for
people with diabetes.
    RC661.A1C34 1999
    616.4'62061—dc21
                                                     99-23163
                                                           CIP

101 MEDICATION TIPS FOR PEOPLE WITH DIABETES

▼

TABLE OF CONTENTS

For our patients, who are our inspiration.
Thank you for teaching us about the realities
of managing diabetes on a daily basis.

PREFACE

▼

If you have type 2 diabetes, you probably take more medications for chronic conditions than anyone you know. This is because along with your diabetes, you may also be dealing with high blood pressure, high cholesterol levels, heart disease, pain, impotence, depression, nausea, and infection. If you are a woman, you can add the use of oral contraceptives or hormone replacement therapy.

The recent introduction of many new drugs for diabetes has expanded the choices you and your doctor have to help manage your blood glucose levels and treat any of your other symptoms. These drugs work in different ways than drugs that have been available for years, and many of them can be used in combination with each other. You may also be taking a variety of vitamin and mineral supplements to improve your health and glucose control.

If you take multiple medications (called "polypharmacy"), your potential for drug-drug and drug-disease interactions is increased. You may feel confused about your complex drug regimen and need clarification on how, when, and why to take each medication. You may be in this for the long haul, taking many of these medications for months or years. It's crucial that you get your questions answered.

As pharmacists who work with people attempting to manage their diabetes on a daily basis, we appreciate how complex drug therapy can be. Even more challenging, we realize that each person brings a unique set of circumstances to be kept in mind when planning a safe and effective drug regimen. Due to the natural progression of type 2 diabetes over time, everybody's medication plan needs constant reevaluation for appropriateness. We also are keenly aware that each day brings new information about drugs and how they should best be used.

People with diabetes, their friends, and their families have asked us many questions about their drug therapy over the years. When we talked with these people about how they were using their medications, we discovered many misconceptions and gaps in information. The questions and tips in this book are a result of our combined experiences spanning many years. We invite you to send us your comments and feedback on this first edition, as well as your own medication questions so we can answer them in future editions.

We hope that after reading this book, you will become smarter consumers and users of drug therapy. It is our intent to provide you with information to help you become an active member of your health care team, maximize your diabetes management, and stay well!

Betsy A. Carlisle, PharmD
Lisa A. Kroon, PharmD
Mary Anne Koda-Kimble, PharmD, CDE

Chapter 1
GENERAL INFORMATION ABOUT MEDICATIONS USED TO TREAT DIABETES

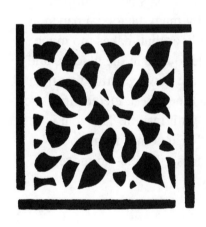

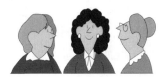

I have many friends and relatives with type 2 diabetes and none of us is being treated with the same medications. Some of us take no medication at all, others of us are on a single medication, and some of us are taking two medications. Two people I know are now using insulin injections. Why are there so many differences in the way we are treated?

▼
TIP:

With type 1 diabetes, the treatment is very straightforward. Because your pancreas no longer produces insulin, you must inject insulin. The treatment of type 2 diabetes is not as simple, because this type of diabetes is caused by many factors: a pancreas that does not produce enough insulin, a liver that makes too much glucose, or muscle cells that are not able to take in the glucose and use it for energy. Different medications are now available that treat these different causes of diabetes. Sometimes these medications are used in combination with each other or with insulin. The goal is to get enough insulin in your body—whether it comes from your pancreas with the help of medications or is injected—to move glucose into your cells to use as energy.

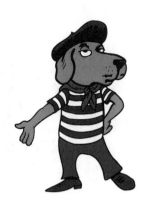

*W*hat medications are available to treat
type 2 diabetes?

▼
TIP:

There are currently six classes or groups of medications available to treat type 2 diabetes. The table below describes the medications in each class. Generally, medications in the same class are not used together because they have the same effect.

Medication Class	Generic Name	Brand Name
Alpha-glucosidase Inhibitors	Acarbose	Precose
	Miglitol	Glyset
Biguanides	Metformin	Glucophage
Meglitinides	Repaglinide	Prandin
Sulfonylureas	Glimepiride	Amaryl
	Glipizide*	Glucotrol
	Glyburide*	DiaBeta
		Glynase
		Micronase
	Tolbutamide	Orinase
	Tolazamide	Tolinase
	Chlorpropamide	Diabinese
	Acetohexamide	Dymelor
Thiazolidinediones**	Troglitazone	Rezulin
Insulin	Insulin	Several

*Available generically.

** Pioglitazone (Actos) and Rosiglitazone (Avandia) will be reviewed by the FDA in 1999.

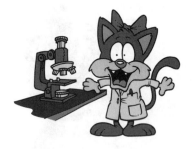

How do the medications listed on page 3 work to lower my blood glucose?

▼
TIP:

All of these medications work differently. Their main site of action in the body and the way in which they lower blood glucose is described in the table below.

Medication Class	Site of Action	Action
Alpha-glucosidase Inhibitors (e.g., Acarbose, Miglitol)	Digestive system	Slows the breakdown of starches to glucose. Slows the entry of glucose into the bloodstream after a meal.
Biguanides (e.g., Metformin)	Liver, muscle	Decreases glucose production by the liver.
Meglitinides (e.g., Repaglinide)	Pancreas	Stimulates insulin release by the pancreas in response to a meal.
Sulfonylureas (e.g., Glyburide or Glipizide)	Pancreas	Stimulates insulin release by the pancreas.
Thiazolidinediones (e.g., Troglitazone)	Muscle, liver, fat cells	Enhances glucose uptake by the muscle.

*A*re oral medications for type 2 diabetes the same as insulin?

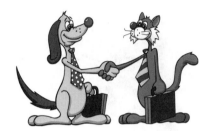

▼
TIP:

No. Oral medications are used to help your pancreas release more insulin or help your own body's insulin work better in lowering your blood glucose. Therefore, you must have a pancreas that releases insulin for almost all of these medications to work (the exception is troglitazone, which works well with insulin injections). Over time, some people with type 2 diabetes are no longer able to produce any insulin from their own pancreas and must be treated with insulin injections.

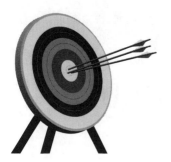

*D*o all medications used to treat type 2 diabetes work equally well?

▼
TIP:

No. Because the medications used to treat type 2 diabetes differ in the way that they work, they also have different abilities (called potency or strength) to lower your blood glucose. As a general rule, the sulfonylureas, meglitinides, and biguanides are more potent in lowering blood glucose than are the thiazolidine-diones or alpha-glucosidase inhibitors when used as single agents.

Medication Class	Decreases Fasting Blood Glucose by:*	Decreases HbA$_{1c}$ by:*
Alpha-glucosidase Inhibitors (e.g., Acarbose, Miglitol)	10–20 mg/dl	0.5–1.0%
Biguanides (e.g., Metformin)	50–70 mg/dl	1.5–1.7%
Meglitinides (e.g., Repaglinide)	50–70 mg/dl	1.5–1.7%
Sulfonylureas (e.g., Glipizide or Glyburide)	50–70 mg/dl	1.5–1.7%
Thiazolidinediones (e.g., Troglitazone)	40 mg/dl	0.8–1.2%

*Each person will respond differently.

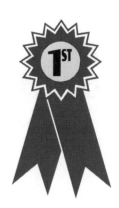

*I*s there a "best" medication to treat
diabetes?

▼
TIP:

S ometimes. There are many factors that help you and your doctor
decide which is the best medication for you. People with type 2
diabetes who are overweight often release adequate amounts of
insulin from their pancreas, but their muscle and fat cells are unable
to respond normally, and their liver manufactures large amounts of
excess glucose. For these people, metformin (Glucophage) may be a
good choice for initial therapy because it is very effective and
doesn't cause weight gain. Patients who have insufficient amounts of
insulin may respond to the use of sulfonylureas. Other people may
have problems with their blood glucose rising immediately
following meals. Acarbose (Precose) or repaglinide (Prandin) may
be good choices for these people. These factors, along with your
current blood glucose levels and the potency (strength) of the
different medications, help you and your doctor select the most
appropriate medication for you. While there may be several possible
medications to control your blood glucose, other factors, such as the
cost of the medication, the number of times per day you have to take
it, and possible side effects, also help determine which medication is
the best for you.

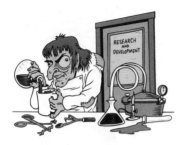

How will I know if my medication is working?

▼
TIP:

By testing your blood glucose. The American Diabetes Association recommends a target blood glucose level between 80 and 120 milligrams per deciliter (mg/dl). Another measure of overall blood glucose control over the past 2 to 3 months is the glycosylated hemoglobin value or hemoglobin A1c (HbA_{1c}). This value should be less than 7% if the upper normal value at your laboratory is 6% (normal values vary from 4% to 6% at different laboratories). It is difficult to tell whether your medication is working without these laboratory tests or without testing your blood glucose values at home. Many people have few or mild symptoms that warn them of high blood glucose concentrations and are surprised when they are told they have diabetes. Some people may notice that their energy levels are increased or that they urinate less frequently after they have been placed on medication.

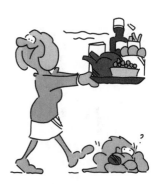

I have controlled my diabetes with diet, but my doctor recently prescribed a medication. Do I still need to follow my diet?

▼
TIP:

Absolutely. The very first step in the treatment of type 2 diabetes is diet combined with exercise to achieve and maintain your desired body weight. Medications are added to diet and exercise therapy when your blood glucose levels exceed the recommended goals. Although some people are able to control their blood glucose and avoid taking medication by following a diet and getting regular exercise, most will eventually require the help of medications as well. Typically, a single medication is added to your diet, using the smallest dose that will help you achieve the desired blood glucose range. All medications (including insulin) work best when you follow dietary guidelines designed by a registered dietitian. By following your diet, you may be able to control your diabetes with low doses of a single medication. It is worthwhile to keep your medication plan as simple as you can for as long as possible.

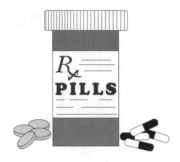

Why am I taking two different medications to treat my diabetes?

▼
TIP:

Two medications (this is called combination therapy) are used to treat type 2 diabetes when the highest dose of a single medication no longer keeps blood glucose values within the desired range. Using two medications that work in different ways to lower your blood glucose often means you can take lower doses of each medication and possibly avoid side effects. Combination therapy can also delay the need for insulin injections for some people.

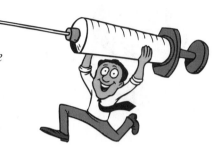

*M*y doctor warned me that I am
taking the highest possible dose
of glyburide and that I may have to
inject insulin in the future. I am
extremely afraid of needles. Is there
any way I can avoid insulin therapy?

▼
TIP:

It depends. There may be other treatment options you can ask for
to delay the need for insulin therapy. Studies show that when you
add a medication that lowers your blood glucose in a different way
to your plan, you might be able to lower your blood glucose further.
Taking a combination of medications and faithfully following your
diet and exercise program may help delay the need for insulin
therapy. Over time, however, the pancreas of many people with
type 2 diabetes stops producing insulin. At this point, they must
inject insulin to lower their blood glucose levels. Some people inject
a small dose of insulin at bedtime while continuing to take their
medication during the day. While it is normal to be afraid of
needles, you might be surprised to realize that the injections are
relatively painless. You'll inject insulin into the fat layer beneath
your skin (where there are fewer nerve endings) using very short
and thin (referred to as fine gauge) needles. Proper training on
injection techniques will help your anxiety and discomfort and helps
you adapt to insulin therapy quite easily.

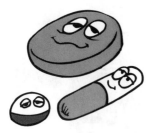

I am now taking two different medications to treat my diabetes, but my blood glucose keeps getting higher. Can I avoid injecting insulin by taking three different medications to treat my diabetes?

▼
TIP:

It's possible that you can. However, because many of the medications available to treat type 2 diabetes are still relatively new and have not been in use for a long time, there is not a lot of information about the proper use of three different medications in combination. Also, the cost of the triple therapy and the increased potential for drug side effects and interactions must be considered. You and your doctor must weigh the benefits and risks in deciding whether triple therapy or insulin injections is the best way to treat your diabetes.

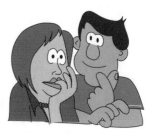

I have a friend with type 2 diabetes who takes insulin injections and tests her blood glucose at home. I am taking a combination of glyburide and metformin. No one ever told me to test my blood glucose. Should I be checking my blood glucose at home too?

▼
TIP:

Yes. Performing blood glucose measurements at home by using a device called a blood glucose meter will tell you whether or not your diabetes is in good control on a daily basis. Home testing gives you valuable information on the effect of diet, exercise, stress, or illness on your blood glucose. The results of home blood glucose testing also help your doctor adjust your current medication regimen. Home testing is easy, although insurance plans do vary in their coverage of blood glucose testing supplies such as test strips, lancet devices, and lancets. The bottom line is that all patients who have access to a meter and are capable of obtaining accurate results should perform blood glucose testing at home to achieve and maintain good glucose control.

Chapter 2
HOW TO GET THE
MOST OUT OF YOUR
ORAL MEDICATIONS

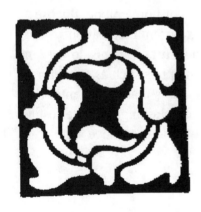

If I forget to take my medication, should I take two pills for the next dose?

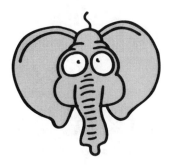

▼
TIP:

As a general rule, you can take a missed dose of any medication as soon as you remember it. However, if you forget to take a dose and it is almost time for your next scheduled dose, skip the missed dose and go back to your regular dosing schedule. Do **not** take a double dose. There are some exceptions to this rule when it comes to medications used to treat your diabetes. If you miss a dose of repaglinide (Prandin), taking the dose between meals could result in a low blood glucose reaction. Therefore, you should not take a missed dose of repaglinide between scheduled meal times. If you miss a dose of acarbose (Precose) or miglitol (Glyset), you should resume your usual regimen at the next scheduled meal, since its action relies on slowing the absorption of high-starch foods.

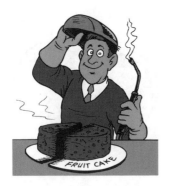

During the holidays when I know I will be eating more, can I increase the amount of medication I am taking to keep my blood glucose under control?

▼
TIP:

Unlike insulin therapy where the amount of insulin can be adjusted to match the meal size, it is very difficult to determine how to adjust an oral medication in a similar manner (a possible exception is repaglinide—ask your doctor). Trying to increase the dose of your diabetes medication during the holidays may result in a low blood glucose reaction. A better idea would be to try to stay on your prescribed diet as much as possible and increase the frequency of your home blood glucose testing to be able to detect any significant elevations in your blood glucose levels.

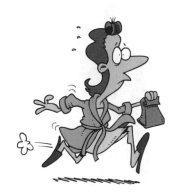

Should I take my medication on an empty stomach or with food?

▼
TIP:

Generally, all of the medications used to treat type 2 diabetes can be taken without regard to a full or empty stomach. However, there are some exceptions.

- Acarbose (Precose) and miglitol (Glyset) should be taken with the first bite of a meal for maximum benefit.
- Metformin (Glucophage) should be taken with meals to minimize stomach upset.
- Troglitazone (Rezulin) should be taken with meals to enhance the amount of medication that is taken up by your intestines into the bloodstream.
- Repaglinide (Prandin) should be taken with meals for maximum benefit and to avoid low blood glucose.

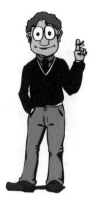

When I refilled my prescription for glipizide, I noticed that the label says to take it 30 minutes before my meals, but sometimes I forget and take it after I eat. Will my medication still work?

▼
TIP:

While some manufacturers suggest taking glipizide 30 minutes before a meal, it has not been proven that this makes any significant difference in the effect of the medication on lowering your blood glucose level. Therefore, you should take your medication as soon as you remember it (see page 15).

*I*s there a best time of the day to take my
medication?

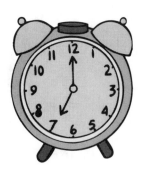

▼
TIP:

This depends upon how many times of the day you are supposed
to take it. If you take once-daily medications with the same
meal each day, you're less likely to forget to take them. It's best to
take twice-daily medications with breakfast and your evening meal.
Repaglinide (Prandin), acarbose (Precose), and miglitol (Glyset)
should generally be taken three times daily with meals. Metformin
(Glucophage) should be taken with meals, whether taken two or
three times daily.

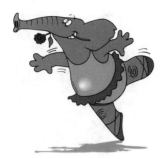

I would like to start an exercise program. Do I need to adjust the dose of my medication if I exercise?

▼
TIP:

During exercise, glucose can enter the muscles without the help of insulin. Because of this, people who exercise vigorously may experience low blood glucose during or immediately following exercise. Exercise also can enhance your body's ability to use glucose. If you inject insulin, you can adjust your insulin dose based on your blood glucose levels before and after exercise. However, there are no such guidelines for adjusting oral medications. Since you are just starting an exercise program, it's important for you to measure your blood glucose levels before and after you exercise. If regular exercise causes a substantial and sustained drop in your daily blood glucose levels or a significant weight loss, the daily dosage of your medication may need to be decreased by your doctor.

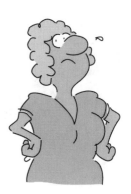

My mother is 70 years old and has just been diagnosed with type 2 diabetes. Her doctor wants to start her on a medication. Is this really necessary at her age?

▼
TIP:

It may be, since diabetes in the elderly can lead to serious complications such as stroke and eye disease if left untreated. Although it may take years for these conditions to develop, your mother may live another 20 years. Diet and exercise are the initial steps in treatment. Her doctor will carefully consider other medical conditions your mother may have before selecting the best medication for her, and will prescribe the smallest effective dose. The doctor will also review any other medications your mother is using to avoid possible drug interactions. Since kidney and liver function can decline with age, her doctor will order regular blood tests to monitor any need to alter your mother's dose of medication.

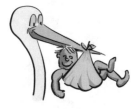

I missed my menstrual cycle and may be pregnant. Will my diabetes medications harm my baby?

▼
TIP:

If you think you may be pregnant, it's important to make an appointment with your doctor immediately so that he or she can evaluate the safety of taking your oral medications. Be sure to tell your doctor if you are planning to become pregnant. Your doctor may advise you to take insulin during your pregnancy. Close control of your blood glucose by using insulin injections during your pregnancy reduces the chance of your baby gaining too much weight, having birth defects, or having high or low blood glucose. Once you have delivered your baby and have stopped nursing, you should be able to discontinue insulin therapy and return to taking your oral medications. If you are already using insulin, the amount of insulin you will need to control your blood glucose will change during and after pregnancy. Insulin does not pass into breast milk and will not affect a nursing infant. However, you may need less insulin while breastfeeding than the dose you were using before your pregnancy.

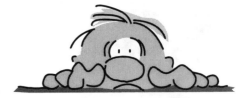

I was told my kidney function is beginning to decline. Will this affect my medication?

▼
TIP:

Your kidneys play an important role in removing medications from your body. Thus, the effect of oral medications or insulin on lowering your blood glucose may be increased because they stay in your bloodstream longer. If this is the case, you may need a smaller dose to control your blood glucose. Laboratory tests such as blood samples and urine collections can be performed to measure how well your kidneys are working. The oral medication of most concern with reduced kidney function is metformin, because of the increased risk for lactic acidosis (high amounts of lactic acid in the blood; see page 36). Certain medications you may be taking for other medical conditions may also slow down the removal of your diabetes medications by your kidneys, so be sure and tell your doctor about anything else you are taking.

I was referred to a heart doctor who gave me a medication called digoxin for heart failure. She told me she would have to change my diabetes medication from metformin to glyburide. Why?

▼
TIP:

Patients with congestive heart failure may be at greater risk for developing lactic acidosis (high amounts of lactic acid in the blood; see page 36) from metformin therapy. The reason for this is that people with heart failure cannot pump blood throughout the body as effectively. This means blood flow to your kidneys is reduced and the amount of metformin in your body may begin to accumulate. Larger amounts of lactic acid may be produced in people who have high amounts of metformin in their bloodstream and also by people who have heart failure. Because rare reports of lactic acidosis in patients with heart failure have been documented, the manufacturer of metformin warns against using this medication in patients with congestive heart failure requiring treatment with medications such as digoxin (Lanoxin), furosemide (Lasix), or captopril (Capoten).

I am allergic to sulfa antibiotics such
as Bactrim. Am I more likely to be
allergic to any of the medications used
to treat diabetes?

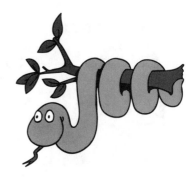

▼
TIP:

It's possible that people with allergies to sulfonamide-type
medications such as sulfa antibiotics or thiazide diuretics (water
pills) develop allergies when using sulfonylurea medications such as
glyburide. Although cases of cross-reactivity (actually developing an
allergy from a sulfonylurea) are rare, it would be better for you to
use a different medication than a sulfonylurea, if you can use one
that is as effective. Talk to your doctor to weigh the benefits and
risks.

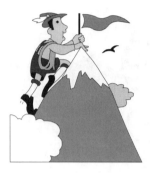

Both my friend and I take glyburide. She takes a 5-mg tablet two times daily and I take two 5-mg tablets once daily in the morning. Which is the better way to take this medication?

▼
TIP:

The number of times a medication is given during the day is based upon something called the "half-life" of the medication. This term refers to the amount of time it takes for about one-half of the medication to be removed from your body. When glyburide was first introduced to the market, it was thought that its half-life was only a few hours and that its effect lasted approximately 12 hours. Thus, glyburide was given twice daily. Now that glyburide has been used extensively in many people, it has been determined that its effect lasts 24 hours or longer. That means it can be given once a day. Whether you take glyburide once or twice daily makes no difference in its ability to lower your blood glucose; however, most people find taking glyburide once daily is easier to remember.

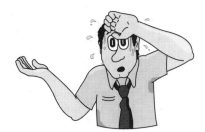

I have been taking 20 mg of glipizide (Glucotrol) two times daily. My doctor just added metformin (Glucophage) to my therapy. I've read that this medication does not cause low blood glucose reactions. Is this true?

▼
TIP:

Yes, but only when metformin is used by itself. You can divide the oral medications currently available to treat type 2 diabetes into two groups: Group #1, hypoglycemic agents such as the sulfonylureas (Glucotrol), repaglinide (Prandin), and insulin; and Group #2, antihyperglycemic agents such as metformin (Glucophage), troglitazone (Rezulin), and acarbose (Precose) or miglitol (Glyset). Group #2 medications lower blood glucose but do not carry a risk for causing low blood glucose reactions (hypoglycemia) when used by themselves. However, when Group #2 medications are used in combination with Group #1 medications, the risk of hypoglycemia increases. Therefore, as your final dose of metformin is determined, you should monitor yourself for symptoms of hypoglycemia (you may sweat, feel nervous, or tremble) and report any of them to your doctor. Also, perform more frequent self-monitoring of blood glucose.

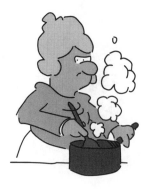

I have been taking 850 mg of metformin twice daily with meals. Now my doctor has added repaglinide (Prandin) to my therapy, and I was told not to take this new medication if I skip a meal. If I do skip a meal, should I also skip my dose of metformin?

▼
TIP:

No. Because repaglinide lowers blood glucose very quickly (usually within 1 hour after taking it), you should only take repaglinide with meals to avoid hypoglycemia. In contrast, metformin does not cause hypoglycemia when taken by itself, so you should still take it.

Chapter 3
COMMON SIDE EFFECTS
OF ORAL MEDICATIONS

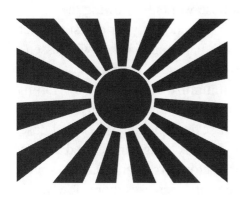

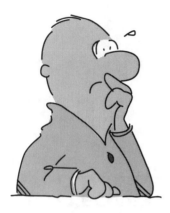

I am taking acarbose and have been experiencing gas, cramps, and diarrhea. Could my medication be causing these symptoms?

▼
TIP:

Yes. Stomach upset, gas, and diarrhea can occur in people taking acarbose. This is because acarbose works by slowing the digestion of carbohydrates, and their presence in your digestive tract causes these symptoms. Your stomach pain and diarrhea will lessen with time and usually disappear. However, your symptoms of gas may not go away entirely. You can minimize these effects by starting with very low doses of acarbose, such as 25 mg once daily, and increasing the dose very slowly over several months. The usual dose is 50 mg with each meal, although up to 100 mg can be used. If you are in a lot of discomfort, ask your doctor if you can decrease your dose of acarbose and make any necessary increases more slowly.

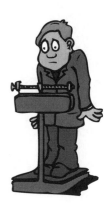

*A*fter my doctor started me on glyburide, my blood glucose got better, but I have gained 8 pounds. Is this caused by my medication?

▼
TIP:

A long with better glucose control, people taking glyburide or other sulfonylureas often experience weight gain. This is because these medications stimulate insulin release from the pancreas. That means less glucose is lost in the urine. Also, high insulin levels in the bloodstream can stimulate your appetite and promote food storage as fat. You may feel more hungry and ultimately gain weight—sometimes up to 4 to 8 pounds. A significant amount of weight gain can cause you to need a larger dose of medication to control your blood glucose. To avoid this problem, you should continue to follow your prescribed meal plan and be alert for any increased appetite or subsequent weight gain.

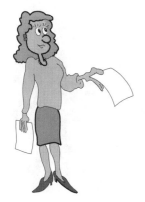

My doctor has given me a prescription for troglitazone (Rezulin). What are the side effects of this medication?

▼
TIP:

Troglitazone is one of the newer medications available for the treatment of type 2 diabetes. It works by improving the ability of your muscle to respond to your body's own insulin or insulin that you may be injecting. Troglitazone is taken once a day with a meal, usually with breakfast, and is generally well tolerated. Some side effects you may experience include symptoms of hypoglycemia and weight gain. Rarely, this medication has been associated with liver problems (see page 35). You can help monitor your liver function in between your monthly blood tests by immediately reporting to your doctor any unusual symptoms of nausea, vomiting, fatigue, or dark urine. For women with polycystic ovary disease, troglitazone can cause menstrual periods to resume. If you are taking an oral birth control pill in addition to troglitazone, the dose of estrogen in your birth control pill may need to be increased, so check with your doctor first.

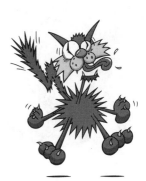

I sometimes feel shaky, nervous, and sweaty. Is this a side effect from my medication?

▼
TIP:

Possibly, especially if you are taking any medications in the sulfonylurea class, repaglinide (Prandin), or insulin. These symptoms are typical warning signals from your body that your blood glucose is dropping below a normal level and you are experiencing hypoglycemia. Because your brain always needs a certain concentration of glucose in your bloodstream to function, these symptoms generally occur when blood glucose values fall below 70 mg/dl. However, the exact concentration at which these warning symptoms occur varies from person to person. While the reason you are having these symptoms could be from taking too much medication, other possible causes include a skipped meal, extra exercise, a drug interaction between your diabetes medication and another medication, or a change in your kidney or liver function. It is very important to recognize what these symptoms mean so that you can appropriately treat your hypoglycemia (see page 34). You also need to figure out what caused the hypoglycemia so you can prevent it next time. If you have frequent hypoglycemia, it is important to notify your health care provider, since your medication dose may have to be reduced.

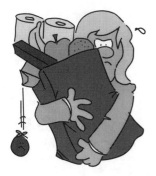

Should I buy glucose tablets to treat my hypoglycemia?

▼
TIP:

Not necessarily. Hypoglycemia should be treated with 10 to 15 grams of a quickly absorbed carbohydrate (glucose or starch). Examples of food sources containing 10 to 15 grams of carbohydrate include 1/2 cup orange juice, 1/3 cup apple juice, two teaspoonfuls of sugar (or 2 cubes), or 5 to 6 pieces of Lifesavers candy. Unfortunately, many people over-treat hypoglycemia by ingesting large amounts of glucose (for example, 1 or 2 candy bars) which results in hyperglycemia (high blood glucose levels). Because glucose tablets are a pre-measured source of glucose (5 grams of glucose per tablet), you may find them easier to use. You also may find it convenient to carry glucose tablets with you when you are working or traveling.

My doctor has prescribed troglitazone (Rezulin) for my diabetes, but told me I will need to have frequent blood tests to check my liver's ALT level. What is this?

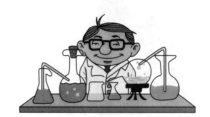

▼
TIP:

Troglitazone (Rezulin) can cause severe liver damage in rare instances (about 1 in 100,000 people). Although this side effect is rare and usually reversible, it is potentially quite serious. Your doctor will run tests to evaluate your liver function before prescribing the drug, once each month for the first 8 months of therapy, and bimonthly for the next 4 months. Thereafter, testing can occur less frequently. When the liver is damaged by medications, a substance called alanine aminotransferase (often abbreviated as ALT) is released into the bloodstream. In most cases, ALT levels return to normal when you stop taking the medication. Therefore, it is very important to keep your appointments to have your ALT level checked. Any symptoms of nausea, abdominal pain, fatigue, or yellowing of your skin should also be reported immediately to your doctor, since these symptoms could also indicate a problem with your liver.

I read that metformin (Glucophage) could cause lactic acidosis. What is this and how would I know if I had it?

▼
TIP:

Lactic acid is a substance that is normally produced by your body in small amounts and removed by your liver and kidneys. Lactic acidosis occurs when this substance builds up in the bloodstream. The risk of developing lactic acidosis is greater if you have other health problems, such as heart failure and lung, kidney, or liver problems. If you have any of these health problems or if you drink alcohol heavily, you probably shouldn't take metformin. Otherwise, you are at a very low risk for developing lactic acidosis from metformin. You should, however, contact your doctor immediately if you suddenly develop diarrhea, fast and shallow breathing, muscle pain or cramping, tiredness, weakness, or unusual sleepiness. These can be symptoms of lactic acidosis. You should also let your doctor know if you get the flu or any illness that results in severe vomiting, diarrhea, and/or fever, or if your intake of fluids becomes significantly reduced. This is because severe dehydration can affect your kidney or liver function and increase your risk of lactic acidosis from metformin.

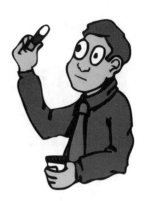

I'm going to have an X ray of my kidneys and was told to stop taking my metformin. Why?

▼
TIP:

Special X-ray tests that require the injection of a dye often cause your kidneys to be temporarily less efficient in clearing lactic acid and other substances from the body. To lessen the risk for lactic acidosis during such a procedure, metformin is stopped before the X ray and restarted about 48 hours afterwards. Before restarting your metformin, your doctor may advise a blood test to make sure that your kidneys are working normally again.

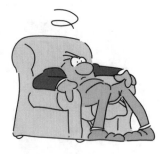

Since I have started taking metformin (Glucophage), I have experienced stomach cramps and diarrhea. Should I stop taking my medication?

▼
TIP:

No. Stomach upset and diarrhea occur commonly during the first two weeks of beginning metformin therapy and usually disappear after a few weeks. Taking each metformin dose with a meal can help reduce stomach discomfort. However, if you have severe discomfort or these side effects do not go away over time, you should contact your doctor. You may need your current dose of metformin lowered or you may need to stop taking metformin, either temporarily or permanently.

I am taking repaglinide (Prandin) for my diabetes. Does this medication have any side effects?

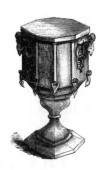

▼
TIP:

The most common side effects reported with the use of repaglinide (Prandin) are hypoglycemia and weight gain. Hypoglycemia can be avoided by taking repaglinide with meals. If you skip a meal, you should skip your dose of repaglinide. Mild weight gain from repaglinide occurs in people being newly treated for diabetes, but it usually does not occur in people being switched from a previous sulfonylurea, such as glyburide, to repaglinide therapy.

Chapter 4
GENERAL INFORMATION ABOUT THE USE OF INSULIN IN TYPE 2 DIABETES

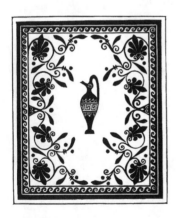

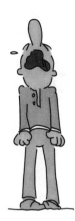

*M*y *doctor recently switched me from taking two different medications for my diabetes to insulin therapy. Does this mean my diabetes is getting worse?*

▼
TIP:

Not necessarily, but it may be changing. In the early phases of diabetes, the pancreas of people with type 2 diabetes has a greater ability to make insulin than in the later stages of diabetes. Therefore, medications that stimulate the pancreas to make more insulin or enhance the action of insulin work better in people who have had diabetes for fewer than 10 to 15 years. As years go by, insulin levels decline and it becomes necessary to supplement the insulin made by the pancreas with insulin injections. Other possible explanations for rising blood glucose levels include weight gain, a decline in your activity or exercise level, taking your medication irregularly, illness, or emotional stress. Depending on your glucose level and other medical conditions, insulin may be needed, either temporarily or permanently.

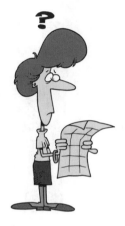

A friend of mine was recently switched from two different oral medications to insulin therapy alone. My doctor added a single injection of insulin at bedtime to my glipizide (Glucotrol). Why didn't my doctor add another kind of medication to my glipizide instead?

▼

TIP:

There are no "recipes" for treating diabetes, because every person's circumstance is unique. When people with type 2 diabetes begin to respond poorly to a combination of oral medications, some diabetes doctors have them discontinue all oral medications and start insulin therapy, because they believe failure to respond to medications means that the pancreas is no longer producing enough insulin. Others choose instead to add a single dose of insulin at bedtime to a single oral medication, because they believe that the pancreas can still release insulin with the help of an oral medication when food is eaten. (However, the pancreas may not be able to make enough insulin to stop glucose production by the liver during the night. This could result in a very high blood glucose level first thing in the morning, making it more difficult for oral medications to maintain reasonable blood glucose levels throughout the day.) Both methods can work depending on the patient.

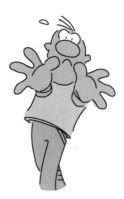

I am now taking the highest doses of glyburide (e.g., DiaBeta) and metformin (Glucophage). My blood glucose level continues to rise and my doctor has told me I will most likely need to begin insulin injections. Are there any other medications I can take to avoid this?

▼
TIP:

Maybe. You can try to delay insulin therapy through more rigorous attention to diet and exercise, or perhaps by adding yet another oral medication. However, currently up to 40% of people with type 2 diabetes must take insulin. Insulin is needed to achieve and maintain blood glucose levels that prevent or slow progression of kidney, eye, and nerve problems. Unfortunately, patients and health care providers alike may have an unreasonable fear of insulin injections. You'll be relieved to hear that insulin injections are virtually painless. This is because needles are now much sharper, thinner, and shorter than before. People who begin insulin therapy commonly report feeling much healthier and more energetic, so it's worth overcoming your fears to try this therapy.

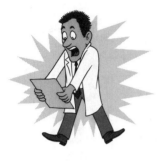

I have been injecting 40 units of NPH insulin each morning. I have been waking up with very high blood glucose levels, and now my doctor has asked me to inject insulin twice daily, in the morning and before supper. Why do I need to do this?

▼
TIP:

The high morning blood glucose values indicate that the effect of a single dose of NPH insulin is not lasting for 24 hours. NPH and lente insulins are both intermediate-acting insulins. They look milky because the insulin is contained in a small particle that takes some time to dissolve and reach the bloodstream once it is injected under the skin. Although these insulins are said to last for 12 to 24 hours, their duration of action will depend on the site of injection and dose. The larger the dose, the longer the duration. However, if a single dose of insulin is increased so that it will last for 24 hours, there is a greater danger of hypoglycemia, especially if you skip a meal during the day. By splitting the injections, very high and very low insulin levels are avoided and it becomes easier to maintain desirable blood glucose levels.

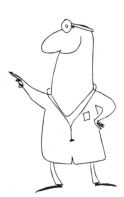

I have been taking two injections of NPH insulin each day. Now my doctor has asked me to begin "mixing" two different kinds of insulin. Why is this necessary?

▼
TIP:

Your doctor is trying to improve your blood glucose control. Although NPH insulin lasts for 12 to 24 hours, it may take 2 to 4 hours to begin working because the insulin particles dissolve so slowly. Because of this, NPH does not work very well to control the blood glucose that rises after you have eaten a meal. For this, you will need an insulin that gets into the body more quickly and has a shorter duration of action. Two types of insulin are used for this purpose: regular insulin and lispro insulin (Humalog). If you look at these insulins, they are clear, like water, because the insulin crystals are dissolved. Thus, they reach the bloodstream much more quickly.

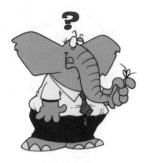

I'm supposed to inject regular insulin 30 minutes before I eat, but it seems I can never predict exactly when that will be. What happens if I take my insulin right when I start eating?

▼
TIP:

You are not alone. Many people find it hard to time their insulin injections in relation to meals. In the ideal world, it is best to have high levels of insulin in the bloodstream at the same time glucose arrives there from a meal you have just eaten. Since it can take 30 to 60 minutes for regular insulin to reach your bloodstream after it is injected, if you wait until mealtime to inject it, you run the risk of hyperglycemia—too much glucose in the bloodstream and not enough insulin to handle it. There is a rapid-acting insulin, lispro (Humalog), that might be a good option for you (see page 47), since it can be injected right before a meal.

I read about an "insulin analog" called lispro (Humalog). What is this?

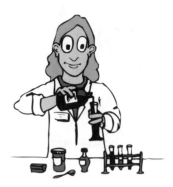

▼
TIP:

This is a rapid-acting insulin that must be taken within 15 minutes before a meal. This feature makes it more convenient than regular insulin for people who are very busy or have unpredictable meal schedules. However, because lispro is very rapid-acting, you must eat within 15 minutes of taking it to avoid a possible low blood glucose reaction. A disadvantage of lispro insulin is that blood glucose can rise again before the next meal because it is so short-acting. To counteract this, some patients mix regular and lispro insulins together. Like regular insulin, lispro insulin can be mixed with longer-acting insulins, but it should be injected soon after the insulins are mixed to make certain the rapid-acting features of this insulin are retained. Lispro is available by prescription only.

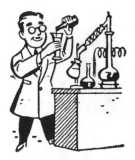

I currently have to mix two different types of insulin. I understand there is a type of insulin that comes already mixed. Can I be switched to this product?

▼
TIP:

Perhaps. It depends on the types of insulin you are mixing and the doses of each. You may have heard of 70/30 and 50/50 products, which are mixtures of intermediate-acting NPH and short-acting regular insulin. The first number refers to the percentage of NPH present and the second number refers to the percentage of regular present in the injected dose. For example, if you inject 10 units of 70/30 insulin, you are taking 7 units of NPH and 3 units of regular insulin. If you currently take NPH and regular insulin in this ratio, it is likely that you could use the premixed product instead with equal results. Premixed insulins can greatly simplify insulin therapy, but they offer very little flexibility in meal planning. This is because the dose of the short-acting insulin, in particular, is strongly determined by the amount of carbohydrate in each meal. In the near future, premixed products containing an intermediate-acting insulin in combination with the rapid-acting insulin lispro (Humalog) will be available.

I *now have to inject insulin three and*
sometimes four times daily. Does this
mean I have a more severe form of
diabetes?

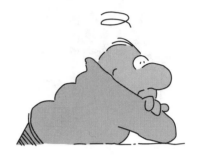

▼
TIP:

N o. This means that your health care provider is trying to deliver
insulin into your bloodstream in a way that mimics the normal
release of insulin from the pancreas. In someone without diabetes,
the pancreas constantly releases just the right amount of insulin to
keep the blood glucose concentration between 70 and 120 mg/dl at
all times. This means that rapid bursts of insulin are released every
time food is eaten in amounts that exactly match the carbohydrate
content of the meal or snack. In between meals, the pancreas
releases very low levels of insulin that prevent the liver from
producing and releasing too much glucose into the bloodstream. So
you use short-acting insulins to provide bursts of insulin before
meals and longer-acting insulins to provide low levels of insulin
between meals. Often, it is possible to achieve better glucose control
over 24 hours with lower total daily doses of insulin by using
smaller doses of insulin injected more frequently. Insulin pumps
deliver insulin by a similar mechanism.

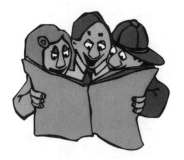

*E*veryone I know who is taking
insulin seems to be on a different
dose. What is a "normal dose" of
insulin?

▼
TIP:

U nfortunately, there is no "normal dose" of insulin. Because
some people are very resistant to the action of insulin, they
require higher doses. Your own insulin requirement may vary, going
up when you are ill, or coming down if you exercise or eat less.
There is a way to evaluate your insulin dose, however. Someone
without diabetes makes about 40 units of insulin a day. You can
estimate the amount of insulin you would need if you didn't have
diabetes by dividing your body weight in pounds by 4. For example,
if you weigh 200 pounds, your estimated need would be about
50 units. Now, add together all your insulin doses to compute your
total daily dose. A dose that is much higher than 50 units suggests
that your body is resistant to insulin action and therefore requires
more than the usual amounts of insulin. A dose that is far lower than
50 units suggests that your body is responsive to insulin and that
your own pancreas is still making and releasing insulin.

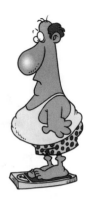

I am taking almost 100 units of insulin a day, yet my diabetes is still not controlled, and I keep gaining weight. Should my insulin dose be increased?

▼
TIP:

Maybe. This is a complicated problem. Obesity and high glucose concentrations decrease the body's ability to release and respond to insulin, so you need to take a higher dose. However, high insulin doses can lead to weight gain (see page 63) and cause hypoglycemia. Your body reacts by releasing hormones that increase blood glucose, and you get rebound hyperglycemia. To avoid this cycle, it is important to step up your efforts to incorporate diet and exercise into your daily care. You should also begin testing your blood glucose levels at home four or more times daily to see if the type of insulin you inject and the number of injections are ideal. It may also be possible to add an oral medication such as metformin (Glucophage) or troglitazone (Rezulin) to your insulin to improve your blood glucose control and decrease your insulin requirements (see page 52).

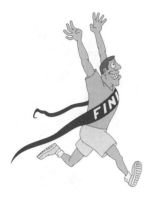

A friend of mine was put on troglitazone (Rezulin) and is now using less insulin. If I took troglitazone, could I stop using insulin?

▼
TIP:

If you take more than 30 units of insulin daily and your diabetes is still not controlled, you may be able to take less insulin and be under better control with troglitazone. Generally, low doses of troglitazone are added to your current dose of insulin while you keep careful track of your blood glucose levels. When your morning (fasting) glucose values are consistently below 120 mg/dl, your total daily insulin dose will be decreased by 10 to 25% to avoid hypo-glycemia. Keep in mind that the primary goal is to improve your blood glucose control, not to lower your insulin dose. In some studies insulin requirements declined by over one-half in 5 out of 10 patients. About one-fourth of patients were able to discontinue insulin altogether, but these were generally those who had been treated with relatively low doses of insulin initially. Several patients were able to decrease the number of insulin injections from 3 to once daily while improving overall glucose control. Therefore, you may not be able to stop using insulin if you add troglitazone to your therapy, but it may decrease the amount of insulin you are using or the number of times you have to inject yourself each day.

I have had type 2 diabetes for 20 years and was started on insulin before many new oral medications were available. Is it possible that I could once again be controlled on an oral medication or a combination of medications?

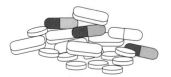

▼
TIP:

Yes. Some diabetes specialists have had success converting people with type 2 diabetes who have been treated with insulin to a combination of oral medications. Generally, these people were switched from medications to insulin during a time when the only oral medications available to treat diabetes were sulfonylureas. Even though there were several different medications within this group, they all had a similar chemical structure and acted in the same way. When people failed to respond to these medications over time, the only other option was insulin. Now there are several new medications that lower blood glucose in different ways. In general, you have the best chance of responding to a combination of oral medications if your total daily insulin requirement is less than 40 units daily, your current blood glucose values are within the target range recommended by the American Diabetes Association (between 80 and 120 mg/dl), and you have had diabetes for less than 15 years.

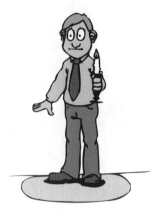

*H*ow *do I know when my insulin is going bad?*

▼
TIP:

It is not always easy to tell if your insulin has lost its potency, but you should make a habit of closely inspecting your insulin vial every time you withdraw your insulin into a syringe. First inspect the insulin for any changes in appearance. Is it discolored? Are there any large particles present in the liquid? Are there salt- or sugar-like crystals on the shoulder of the vial? Has your regular or lispro insulin that is supposed to be clear become cloudy? If any of these visible changes occur, the vial should be discarded. However, keep in mind that other changes may not be observable with the naked eye, so always be alert for any indication that your insulin may not be working as well (such as high blood glucose levels), especially when there are no other explanations. To minimize this possibility, date your vial when you begin using it, store it properly (see page 61), and discard it after 4 weeks, or as recommended by the manufacturer.

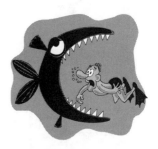

My health insurance company changed the brand of insulin it covers. Is it safe to switch brands?

▼
TIP:

Yes, with a few exceptions. Regular, NPH, lente and ultralente insulins made by different manufacturers have the same potency, onset, and duration of action. However, some products are unique to specific manufacturers and brands. Specific examples include lispro (Humalog) made by Lilly, Humulin 50/50 made by Lilly, and Velosulin made by Novo Nordisk. If you are using lispro (Humalog) as your rapid, short-acting insulin, it should be mixed only with Lilly brands of NPH, lente, or ultralente human insulins. It is not known whether lispro will retain its rapid-acting characteristics if it is mixed with other brands of intermediate- or long-acting insulins.

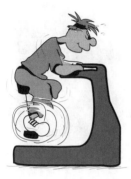

*H*ow does exercise affect my insulin
therapy?

▼
TIP:

Exercise may lower your insulin requirements, and this effect can last for several hours if the exercise is strenuous. Since your body uses less insulin during exercise, your usual dose of insulin can have a greater effect in lowering your blood glucose. Also, if you inject your insulin in an area near a major muscle group such as your thigh, the onset of effect from your insulin may be quicker. Therefore, if you anticipate that your activity level will be substantially increased, you should be alert for signs and symptoms of hypoglycemia and you should take care not to delay or skip a meal. If you are planning to begin a more vigorous exercise plan, work with your health care provider to adjust your insulin doses before beginning your program.

*W*ill I always have to take insulin by
injection?

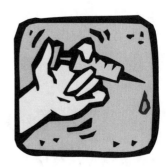

▼
TIP:

Perhaps not. Several groups are studying ways to give insulin as a
nasal spray, an inhaler, or as a drug patch, but there a many
challenges that must be overcome to get enough insulin into the
bloodstream using these methods. Unfortunately, insulin cannot be
taken in pill form, because it is a fragile protein that is destroyed
and digested by the stomach and intestines before it reaches the
blood circulation. Therefore, to get an active form of insulin into the
blood, these organs must be bypassed. Injection is the most direct
way to get precise amounts of insulin into the body. When given as
a nasal spray, up to 3 times the dose of insulin is needed to produce
an effect similar to an injection. Not enough research has been done
on insulin patches.

Chapter 5
HOW TO GET THE MOST
OUT OF YOUR
INSULIN THERAPY

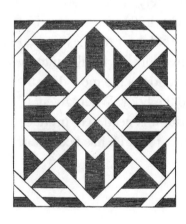

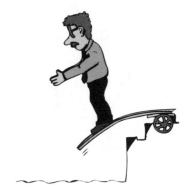

*W*here is the best place to inject my
insulin?

▼
TIP:

There is no "best place" to inject insulin. The abdomen, arms, thighs, and hips may be used. However, many health care practitioners recommend the abdomen as the primary site because it is a large area that is easily reached and insulin gets into the bloodstream quickly. It is also the site least affected by exercise (see page 56). To avoid the development of lumps, you should rotate your insulin injections throughout the abdomen and avoid the area around your belly button (see page 65). If you use various body sites, you should keep the site consistent based on the time of injection. For example, always use the thigh for morning injections, the upper arm for noontime injections, and the abdomen for evening injections. When using these other sites, remember to rotate your insulin injections throughout the area.

My mother has type 2 diabetes that is treated with regular and lente insulin. Because she has poor eyesight and arthritis, I prepare several syringes for her twice weekly and store them in the refrigerator. Is this safe?

▼
TIP:

Yes, if you use a good, clean technique and label the containers in which they are stored with the date of preparation. However, it probably is prudent to premix no more than a week's supply at a time and to discard any unused syringes. You should be aware that when regular insulin is mixed with lente insulin, the action of regular insulin may be slowed and prolonged if the mixture is not used within 15 minutes. If your mother is meeting her glucose control goals, this may not be an issue, but ask her to tell her health care provider that you are preparing her insulin injections in advance. Another alternative is to work with your mother's provider to change from lente to NPH insulin, which is more compatible with regular insulin and does not change its action when mixed together and stored for short periods.

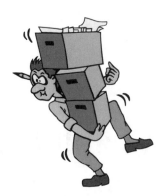

I *don't like injecting cold insulin. Can I store my insulin at room temperature?*

▼
TIP:

Yes. Insulin may be stored at room temperature for 1 month, but it should be kept in a place where the vial will not be exposed to temperature extremes (above 86 degrees or below 40 degrees Fahrenheit). During winter and summer months, this can be accomplished by keeping insulin in an insulated container. Insulin is a delicate protein molecule that can be changed or destroyed by heat, freezing, or too much agitation. Extra insulin that is not in use should be kept in the refrigerator. When you open a new vial, write on the label the date that it is opened or the date that it should be discarded (28 days later). The expiration date printed on the label by the manufacturer signifies the date after which insulin should not be used under ideal, refrigerated storage conditions.

Chapter 6
COMMON SIDE EFFECTS
OF INSULIN

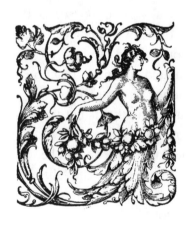

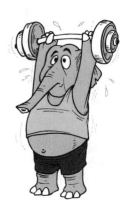

Since I started using insulin 6 months ago, I have gained 10 pounds. I feel frustrated because I have stuck to my diet. Is this weight gain caused by my insulin?

▼
TIP:

Probably. Most people who use insulin gain weight—sometimes up to 15 to 20 pounds. Although the added pounds can be discouraging, they may actually signal better diabetes control. People with poorly controlled diabetes lose tremendous amounts of glucose (and therefore calories) in their urine. However, when blood glucose concentrations fall to less than 180 mg/dl, little or no glucose is spilled into the urine. Also, remember that insulin is a "storage" hormone. It helps the body's cells pick up glucose and other fuels from food and store them for future use. Because producing fat is one of the most efficient ways to store fuel, people taking insulin will tend to gain weight. Weight gain can be minimized by properly adjusting your insulin dose to just the right amount you need to keep your blood glucose levels within the target range without causing too many lows. Low blood glucose levels cause hunger and overeating, and this also may contribute to weight gain.

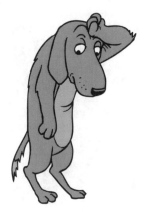

I have night sweats and often wake up in the morning with headaches. Is this related to my insulin?

▼

TIP:

It could be. The symptoms you describe can be caused by hypoglycemia while you are sleeping. You may be injecting too much insulin in relation to your evening food. Or, you may be injecting too much of the wrong type of insulin. People who inject an intermediate-acting insulin such as NPH or lente in the early evening before dinner sometimes experience similar symptoms. These insulins have their most potent action 6 to 10 hours later, which corresponds to the early morning hours when glucose concentrations are normally at their lowest level. Discuss these symptoms with your health care provider. In the meantime, set your alarm for 3:00 A.M. and test your glucose level at that time and again first thing in the morning for several days in a row. You may want to delay the injection of NPH or lente from before your evening meal to bedtime. This shifts the peak action of these insulins to the early morning hours when you will be rising and ready to eat breakfast.

*I have developed lumps on my stomach
where I inject my insulin. Is there anything
I can do about this?*

▼
TIP:

Give the lumps on your stomach a rest from insulin injections. Fat pads and lumps occur when insulin is repeatedly injected into the same place. By carefully rotating your injection sites, you should not have to use the same site more often than every 2 weeks or so. If the lump is in one area of your abdomen, rotate the injections around unaffected areas. If the lumps are all over the abdomen, you should probably begin injecting insulin into your thighs, buttocks, and arms. The lumps you describe are not dangerous or harmful, but some people are troubled by their appearance. When insulin is injected into these lumps, it cannot get into the bloodstream as quickly and this can delay and prolong its action. If you give your abdomen a rest, the lumps may slowly go away after several weeks or months, depending on their size. But if they are large and bothersome, surgical removal may be the only solution.

Chapter 7
MEDICATIONS USED TO TREAT COMPLICATIONS OF DIABETES

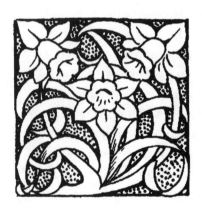

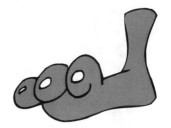

I have developed tingling and burning in both of my feet that seems to get worse at night. Are there medications I can take to treat this problem?

▼
TIP:

You are experiencing symptoms of diabetic neuropathy, a nerve disease caused by chronically high blood glucose levels. Medications used to treat this pain are not always effective. It will help you the most if you normalize your blood glucose levels and quit smoking (if you are a smoker). You can try nonprescription analgesics such as acetaminophen (Tylenol) and ibuprofen (Advil), but you may need prescription medications. Tricyclic antidepressants such as amitriptyline (Elavil) are the most commonly used. Although these medications are traditionally used to treat depression, they can be very effective for pain due to nerve damage. Other antidepressants used are fluoxetine (Prozac) and paroxetine (Paxil). Anti-seizure medications such as phenytoin (Dilantin) and carbamazepine (Tegretol) have also been used to treat neuropathy. A newer anti-seizure medication called gabapentin (Neurontin) is showing promise. Narcotic analgesics such as codeine plus acetaminophen (Tylenol #3) or Vicodin are effective, but unfortunately lose their effectiveness over time. Because they can be addictive, narcotics are usually tried after all of the above medications have failed.

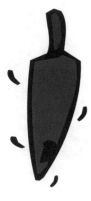

I *have heard there is a "red pepper" cream that will improve the pain in my feet. Can I use it safely?*

▼
TIP:

Yes. A "red pepper" cream is available to treat the pain in your feet caused by nerve disease. The active ingredient is capsaicin, a chemical found in hot chili peppers. When you apply it topically to your feet, it causes a depletion of a body chemical called substance P, which causes the pain. Initially, capsaicin causes substance P to be released from cells, which in turn causes a burning or stinging sensation (similar to how your mouth feels when you eat hot peppers). When capsaicin is applied regularly (3 to 4 times daily for several weeks), substance P is eventually depleted from cells and you'll feel relief from pain. Capsaicin cream can be used safely, but you must be careful to use gloves or to wash your hands thoroughly after application to avoid getting this medication into your eyes. Capsaicin does not work for everybody, but it may be an option for you. It is available without a prescription as a 0.025%, 0.05%, or 0.075% cream or ointment (Zostrix). A prescription strength (0.25%) product is also available (Dolorac).

*M*y *doctor told me I have small amounts of protein in my urine and prescribed an ACE inhibitor for me. I thought this was a medication for high blood pressure. Why do I need to take this?*

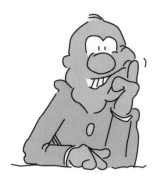

▼
TIP:

The ACE (angiotensin-converting enzyme) inhibitors are used to treat many conditions, including high blood pressure, heart failure, and diabetic kidney disease. Your doctor may have prescribed an ACE inhibitor so that you may benefit from its protective effect on your kidneys. Albumin is a protein that is normally found in the bloodstream but not in the urine. The small amount of albumin in your urine (called "microalbuminuria") is an early signal of kidney damage. Without treatment, microalbuminuria can worsen to a more severe form of kidney disease in 20 to 40% of people with type 2 diabetes. It is important to monitor your blood glucose levels when you start an ACE inhibitor because it will occasionally cause low blood glucose reactions. Other measures that will protect your kidneys include very good control of your blood pressure (aim for less than 130/85 mmHg) and blood glucose levels (70–140 mg/dl).

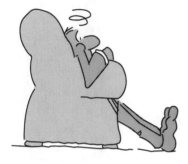

I get full easily and often feel sick and nauseated after I eat. Are there any medications that can help relieve this?

▼
TIP:

The nerve disease seen in people with diabetes can sometimes affect the nerves of the stomach. This is called gastroparesis (or paralysis of the stomach). The stomach doesn't empty food as rapidly, causing an early feeling of fullness or nausea during a meal. Achieving good glucose control is important to help alleviate the symptoms. There are several prescription medications used to help relieve gastroparesis: metoclopramide (Reglan), cisapride (Propulsid), and erythromycin. These medications all increase the stomach's ability to contract and aid in digestion. It is best to try these medications one at a time to see if one of them will work for you.

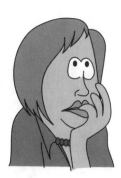

I *am often constipated. Are there any medications that I can take to help with this problem?*

▼
TIP:

The nerve disease seen in people with diabetes can also affect the nerves in the bowel, leading to constipation. Try to increase the amount of fluids and fiber in your diet. However, you should avoid large amounts of juices and drink more water instead in order to prevent fluctuations in your blood glucose levels. You can try laxatives such as psyllium (Metamucil) and methylcellulose (Citrucel). These are bulk-forming laxatives that cause an increase in pressure, leading to contraction of the bowel muscles and defecation. Psyllium tends to cause more gas and cramping than methylcellulose. Stimulant laxatives, such as Ex-lax and senna, are usually effective. However, the bowel can become dependent on them, which means you cannot have a bowel movement without them. Cisapride (Propulsid), a prescription medication that causes the bowel muscles to contract, has also been used. Since many medications can cause constipation, you should ask your pharmacist or doctor to review your list of medications. It may be possible to use an alternative medication or modify the dose to avoid constipation.

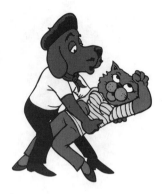

I have increasing difficulty maintaining an erection during intercourse. Are there any medications that can help improve this problem?

▼
TIP:

Yes, depending on the cause of impotence. Men with diabetes can develop impotence, which is defined as the consistent inability to achieve or maintain an erection sufficient for satisfactory performance during intercourse. About 50% of men with diabetes become impotent during their lifetime. The main causes of impotence are decreased blood flow to the penis from plaque deposits in the circulatory system or diabetic nerve disease. Many non-medication approaches are used, including psychotherapy, penile implants or prostheses, and vacuum constriction devices. The FDA-approved medication therapies include alprostadil (Muse) and sildenafil (Viagra). Muse must be injected into the penis or inserted as a pellet into the urethra; Viagra is a tablet that is taken 30 minutes to 4 hours before intercourse. Sildenafil inhibits the breakdown of one of the chemical components involved in an erection and improves intercourse success rates in about 50% of men with diabetes. Side effects are mild and can include facial flushing, headache, and indigestion. Sildenafil cannot be used by men who take nitrates in any form because a dangerous drop in blood pressure can result.

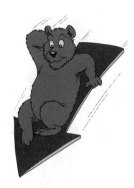

I have high blood pressure. What medication should I take?

▼
TIP:

High blood pressure contributes to the development and worsening of complications due to diabetes. The target blood pressure in people with diabetes is less than 130/85 mmHg, which is slightly lower than the recommended blood pressure for the general population. There are many groups of medications that are effective in lowering blood pressure in people with diabetes. However, because ACE inhibitors also help protect the kidneys, they are often preferred (see page 69). In certain situations, the use of one medication may not be effective enough in lowering the blood pressure, so a second medication will be needed. A group of water pills called thiazide diuretics is very effective in lowering blood pressure when used in combination with ACE inhibitors. A group of calcium channel blockers called nondihydropyridines has been used successfully (another group, the dihydropyridines, is not used for people with diabetes). Examples include diltiazem (Cardizem), verapamil (Calan), and nifedipine (Procardia). Many people with diabetes also take calcium channel blockers for angina pectoris (chest pain) or after a heart attack.

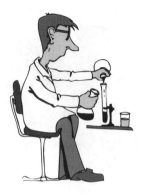

My doctor started me on captopril for my kidney disease and I have developed a dry cough that won't seem to go away. Are there other medications that can be used for my kidneys instead?

▼
TIP:

Yes. Ask your doctor about the calcium channel blockers diltiazem (Cardizem), verapamil (Calan), and nifedipine (Procardia). However, doctors disagree as to how well these drugs will protect your kidneys. Another group of medications called angiotensin receptor II antagonists work similarly to the ACE inhibitors, but do not cause a cough. Examples include losartan (Cozaar), valsartan (Diovan), and Irbesartan (Avapro). Studies are underway to determine whether they too will prevent the worsening of diabetic kidney disease. Some practitioners will try another ACE inhibitor, but typically, once you have developed a cough from one ACE inhibitor, it is unlikely that you will be able to tolerate others. Therefore, switching to an angiotensin receptor II antagonist is probably your best option.

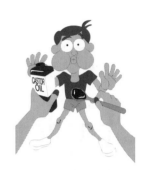

I *feel like I am taking so many medications*
for my heart, cholesterol, high blood
pressure, and diabetes. Do I really need to take
them all?

▼
TIP:

Yes. It is quite common for people with type 2 diabetes to be taking many medications at the same time. This is because people with diabetes often have other conditions, such as high blood pressure, heart disease, high cholesterol or triglycerides, obesity, and insulin resistance. This collection of conditions has been termed Syndrome X or Insulin Resistance Syndrome. It is well known that people with type 2 diabetes don't usually die from the diabetes itself. The major cause of death in people with this type of diabetes is heart disease. Thus, it is very important to treat the conditions that will increase your risk of heart disease, such as high blood pressure, high blood cholesterol levels, diabetes, obesity, and smoking.

Chapter 8
EFFECT OF MEDICATIONS ON DIABETES

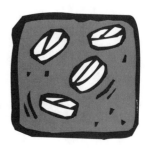

*W*hat are the most common medications
that can increase my blood glucose
levels?

▼
TIP:

A group of steroids called glucocorticoids can significantly raise
your blood glucose by causing insulin resistance. This group
includes medications such as prednisone, hydrocortisone, dexa-
methasone, and cortisol. Glucocorticoids are used to treat a variety
of conditions, such as rheumatoid arthritis, asthma, and severe
allergic reactions. Your blood glucose levels are likely to rise if you
take large doses of these medications as pills or by injection. When
you inhale them or rub them on your skin as an ointment or cream,
they have low potential to increase blood glucose, because very little
of the steroid is absorbed into your bloodstream. Fortunately, the
effect of steroids on blood glucose is usually reversible. Niacin
(nicotinic acid) can also increase blood glucose (see page 83), as
can protease inhibitors (medications used to treat people with
HIV/AIDS). When treating medical conditions with drugs, you and
your doctor must weigh the benefits against the risks of therapy.
Sometimes the benefit gained from treating your condition will
outweigh the risk of increasing your blood glucose. In that case, the
effect on blood glucose can be managed by adjusting your diabetes
treatment plan.

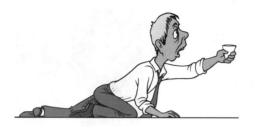

*I*s it OK for me to drink
alcohol? How much can I
drink?

▼
TIP:

The effect of alcohol on blood glucose depends on how much
you drink in what period of time. Large amounts of alcohol over
a short time can cause hypoglycemia by preventing the liver from
making glucose. You can get severe hypoglycemia if you drink
alcohol and take medications that also can cause hypoglycemia,
such as insulin, sulfonylureas, and repaglinide. Unfortunately, the
signs and symptoms of hypoglycemia may not be recognized,
because they can be confused with drunkenness. You are most
vulnerable to this effect if you drink heavily, drink large amounts on
an empty stomach, and do not eat while you are drinking. You
should know that heavy drinking (defined as more than two drinks
daily, every day) can worsen your blood glucose control (one drink
is 12 ounces of beer, 5 ounces of wine, or 1½ ounces of distilled
spirits). If you take chlorpropamide (Diabinese), you may
experience flushing of your face and body while drinking. It is best
to discuss alcohol intake with your physician or dietitian. Keep in
mind that alcohol is a source of calories and needs to be included in
your meal plan.

*I*s it safe for me to take birth control pills, or will they make my diabetes worse?

▼
TIP:

Estrogens and progestins, the two active ingredients found in most birth control pills, will not generally make your diabetes worse. Birth control pills can increase your risk for blood clots if you have peripheral vascular disease (blood circulation problems). However, the doses of estrogen now used in most birth control pills are much lower than doses used in the past, so this problem is not quite as frequent as it used to be. Women who smoke or have diabetes are at an increased risk of developing peripheral vascular disease. To minimize your risk of peripheral vascular disease from birth control pills, use a low-dose estrogen product, keep your blood glucose levels under control, and do not smoke. Women over 35 who have diabetes and smoke should probably not take birth control pills, due to an increased risk of coronary heart disease.

My doctor wants to prescribe estrogen therapy now that I am postmenopausal, but doesn't estrogen increase blood fat levels? I am already taking a medication called Tricor (fenofibrate) for my high triglyceride levels.

▼
TIP:

Women are thought to be protected against heart disease before menopause by their natural estrogen hormones. Unfortunately, if you have diabetes, you are already at a greater risk for heart disease. Because of this, if your cholesterol levels are high, your are probably taking a cholesterol-lowering medication. Estrogen replacement therapy has been shown to increase the good cholesterol (HDL) as well as decrease the bad cholesterol (LDL), which reduces your risk of heart disease. The main concern with the use of estrogen therapy is the increased risk for breast or endometrial cancer. However, the risk of cancer is quite small compared to the anticipated reduction in heart disease risk. You should not be on estrogen if you have a family history of endometrial or breast cancer, clotting disorders, or liver disease. Estrogen replacement can increase triglyceride concentrations by 20%; however, your current dose of fenofibrate should be able to compensate for this potential increase.

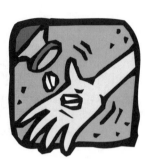

*A*fter I had a heart attack, my doctor put
me on a beta-blocker. I've heard this kind
of medication is bad for someone with
diabetes. Should I take it?

▼
TIP:

Yes. Medications called beta-blockers are commonly prescribed
after a heart attack because people who take them are more
likely to survive 1 year after their first heart attack. The beta-
blockers metoprolol (Lopressor) or atenolol (Tenormin) may be
prescribed for this use. Previously, doctors were warned to use beta-
blockers cautiously in people with diabetes because they might
block or "mask" warning symptoms of hypoglycemia, such as heart
palpitations and shakiness. Beta-blockers can also slow the body's
recovery if hypoglycemia occurs. However, the benefits of
preventing future heart attacks far exceed these risks. If you are
taking medications for diabetes that could cause hypoglycemia and
are started on a beta-blocker following a heart attack, you should
test your blood glucose level more frequently and be aware that your
normal warning symptoms of hypoglycemia may be blunted.
Sweating, a common symptom of hypoglycemia, is not affected by
beta-blockers.

I take a water pill called hydrochlorothiazide for high blood pressure. Doesn't this increase blood glucose levels? Is it OK to take?

▼
TIP:

Hydrochlorothiazide, a thiazide diuretic that is often referred to as a "water pill," can increase your blood glucose by causing insulin resistance. However, the effect on your blood glucose depends on the dose you take. In the past, doses of 25 to 50 mg daily were commonly used to treat high blood pressure. But these days it's more common to take doses as low as 12.5 mg, which are as effective for blood pressure control and have minimal effects on the blood glucose level. The thiazide diuretics have also been shown to elevate blood lipid levels, but this is not a concern if doses are 25 mg per day or lower.

*M*y daily multivitamin contains niacin. I've heard this can cause my blood glucose to rise. Should I stop taking it?

▼
TIP:

No. Niacin, or nicotinic acid, can increase your blood glucose, but at much higher doses than those contained in a multi-vitamin tablet. Niacin is a form of vitamin B3, as is niacinamide (also called nicotinamide). The amount usually contained in these products is 50 to 100 micrograms. People who take niacin to lower their cholesterol levels take 20 to 60 times this amount or 2 to 6 grams daily. These higher amounts usually do increase blood glucose levels.

Chapter 9
NONPRESCRIPTION
MEDICATIONS

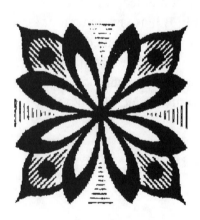

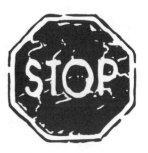

Many medications you can buy without a prescription say "consult with your physician before using if you have diabetes." Should I heed these warnings? Are there any general rules to use when buying medications without a prescription?

▼
TIP:

Yes. Always read the labels carefully. It is important to see if a product contains sugar or alcohol. Look in the "active" and the "inactive" ingredients sections. Use tablets or capsules when possible, since they generally contain less sugar and alcohol compared to liquid products. Avoid combination products, which tend to have hidden ingredients that could potentially be harmful. Some over-the-counter products may have side effects that can be harmful if you have diabetes. Some can increase or decrease your blood glucose. Others may worsen diabetic complications such as nerve or kidney disease. Some have a negative effect on other conditions such as high blood pressure or high blood lipids. Therefore, it is very important to read the labels of these products to see if there are any warnings regarding diabetes, high blood pressure, or heart disease. If such warnings are present, ask your physician or pharmacist if the product is safe for you to take.

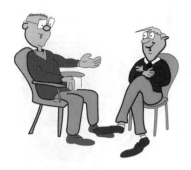

*S*hould I tell my physician if I am
taking any medications I purchased
without a prescription?

▼
TIP:

Yes. Always tell your physician and pharmacist about any over-the-counter products you take. Like all medications, these products can cause harmful side effects, even though you don't need a prescription for them. Your physician and pharmacist can check the product to see if it interacts with any medications you are currently taking or if it could make any of your current medical conditions worse. When telling your physician or pharmacist which over-the-counter medications you are taking, be sure to include dietary supplements, such as vitamins and minerals, and herbal products, including herbal teas.

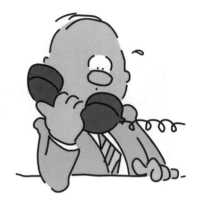

I read a newspaper article indicating that I should take one aspirin every day since I have diabetes. How much aspirin is recommended?

▼
TIP:

The American Diabetes Association (ADA) recommends that people with diabetes who have had a heart attack, undergone heart bypass surgery, or suffered a stroke take an aspirin daily. People who have angina, poor circulation in the legs, a family history of heart disease, high blood pressure, obesity, kidney disease, high blood cholesterol, or who smoke should also take a daily aspirin. People with diabetes who are under the age of 30 and do not have heart disease risk factors or those who have an aspirin allergy, bleed easily, are taking a blood thinner such as warfarin (Coumadin), or have serious liver disease are not advised to take aspirin. The ADA recommends anywhere from 81 mg (equivalent to a "baby" aspirin) up to 325 mg of aspirin daily. The warning labels advising against aspirin use often placed on vials of diabetes medications apply only to large doses of aspirin (for example, 12 tablets daily for arthritis). Always ask your pharmacist to clarify what the warning label on a prescription means.

 *If I take aspirin, should I take a buffered or coated aspirin pill to protect my stomach?*

▼
TIP:

The American Diabetes Association recommends use of an enteric-coated aspirin tablet. The risk of stomach bleeding depends on the amount and for how long you have taken aspirin. Enteric coating allows the aspirin tablet to bypass the stomach so that it dissolves in and is absorbed from the upper intestines. This decreases the chance of indigestion due to direct irritation of the stomach lining. However, because coated aspirin is absorbed into your bloodstream, it can still get back to your stomach lining where it can cause bleeding through another mechanism. Buffered aspirin tablets contain a "buffer" or antacid, which allows the aspirin to dissolve much more quickly. Unfortunately, the amount of antacid contained in each tablet is not likely to protect the stomach lining. Symptoms of a bleeding stomach include a substance that looks like coffee grounds in your vomit, black tarry stools, and a weak or dizzy feeling. Alert your physician if you have any of these symptoms. Many manufacturers use different terms to indicate enteric coating of their aspirin products, such as "safety-coated." Make sure to read the label carefully.

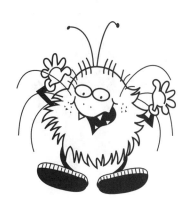

*I have a cold and am terribly
congested. Most cough and cold
products warn against use if you have
diabetes or high blood pressure. I have
both. What general advice can you give
me in selecting a product?*

▼
TIP:

G enerally, you should avoid any product that claims to be a
"nasal decongestant." These work by constricting the blood
vessels in your nose to relieve congestion, but if taken by mouth,
they also can constrict the blood vessels throughout your body,
thereby raising your blood pressure. If your blood pressure is well
controlled, your physician may decide a low dose of decongestant is
safe for you to use. Examples of decongestants are phenylephrine
(Actifed), phenylpropanolamine (Dimetapp), and pseudoephedrine
(Sudafed). These medications can also cause your blood glucose to
rise. Unlike tablet or liquid decongestants, nasal sprays will not
affect your blood glucose because they act locally and little of the
medication reaches the bloodstream. Examples include Afrin and
Dristan nasal sprays. These topical sprays are very effective, but
should be used only occasionally and for no longer than 3 days at a
time to avoid "addicting" your nasal passages. If your congestion is
due to allergies, you can probably take antihistamines.

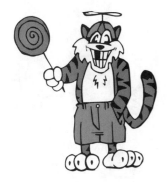

*H*ow important is the sugar content of medication I can buy without a prescription?

▼
TIP:

Not too important. Liquid formulations of nonprescription medications commonly contain sugar in order to make them taste better. Often the amount of sugar is minimal and will not greatly affect your blood glucose levels. Of course, it depends on the amount of nonprescription medication you take and how long you use it. If you notice your blood glucose is greatly affected when taking a product, ask your pharmacist whether a sugar-free formulation is available. If you require an over-the-counter product on a regular basis, consider taking a pill or capsule form if it is available, since the sugar content in these products is minimal.

I have developed a corn on my little toe *as well as some athlete's foot. Can I use medications that do not require a prescription to self-treat my feet?*

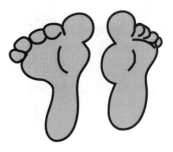

▼
TIP:

It is best not to self-medicate corns, calluses, or blisters on your feet. The salicylic acid used in most products can irritate and damage your skin. You may not detect skin damage early because of decreased sensation in your feet. Furthermore, if an ulcer or infection occurs, healing may be difficult and prolonged because blood flow to your feet may be diminished. Ask your physician or podiatrist to treat and monitor any corns, calluses, or blisters. It is probably safe to treat your athlete's foot, but do let your physician or podiatrist know that you have this condition. You should inspect your feet daily to look for sore, red spots that can turn into blisters and skin cracks that can become infected. If your feet don't improve, inform your physician or podiatrist, since you may need a prescription-strength medication. Be sure to wear well-fitting cotton socks that absorb excess moisture, change your socks daily to avoid reinfecting your feet, and dry your feet well after bathing or showering.

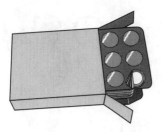

What are the safest medications I can use to treat a headache or fever?

▼
TIP:

Aspirin, nonsteroidal anti-inflammatory agents (NSAIDS), and acetaminophen (Tylenol) can be used to treat a fever and headaches and are all equally effective. Examples of NSAIDS available without prescription include ibuprofen (Advil and Motrin IB), ketoprofen (Orudis KT and Actron), and naproxen (Aleve). Aspirin and NSAIDS are often considered less preferable because of their potential for stomach irritation and kidney toxicity. However, when used for a few days, they are generally safe. In contrast, chronic use of NSAIDS and large doses of aspirin are of particular concern for people with kidney disease, and acetaminophen can be toxic to the liver if taken in high doses. Even with a healthy liver, you should not use more than 4 grams (8 500-mg tablets or capsules) daily of acetaminophen. If you currently have or have had any problems with your kidneys or liver or if your fever persists for longer than 72 hours, contact your health care provider. Check the ingredients labels to make sure the product is safe for people with diabetes. Ask your pharmacist if you have any concerns or, better yet, use a simple analgesic product that contains a single ingredient.

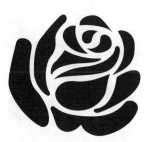

I've had a vaginal yeast infection in the past and I know the symptoms. Can I buy something at the drugstore to treat this problem myself?

▼ TIP:

Vaginal yeast infections may be a sign of poorly controlled diabetes, because organisms thrive in high blood glucose levels. High blood glucose levels also impair the body's ability to fight infection, and the infection itself is a stress factor that makes blood glucose control more difficult. For these reasons, this problem should be brought to your physician's attention. Women with poorly controlled diabetes often do not respond to nonprescription products for vaginal yeast infections and require a prescription antibiotic. Improving your blood glucose control is also important to prevent repeat vaginal yeast infections.

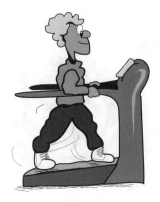

My doctor told me my diabetes would improve if I lost weight. Should I try something like Dexatrim?

▼
TIP:

Several nonprescription products are available for weight loss. While products that provide "bulk" and a feeling of fullness are generally safe to use, many nonprescription products that suppress the appetite contain a drug called phenylpropanolamine. This drug can increase your blood glucose level and blood pressure, both of which are undesirable effects. Some herbal weight-loss products, although called "natural," also contain similar drugs and should be avoided. For example, the herb ma huang or ephedra is the botanical source of ephedrine, which acts like adrenaline, and can have undesirable effects on your blood glucose level, blood pressure, and heart. As you probably know, exercising regularly and eating less are key components to successful and permanent weight loss. If these lifestyle changes are ineffective, you can discuss other options with your physician or dietitian. Although some prescription medications are available, people often gain weight back after they stop taking them. You'll have more luck with a comprehensive, behavioral approach to weight loss.

I read about some special vitamin and mineral supplements for people with diabetes. Do people with diabetes have special needs for vitamins? If so, which ones should I take?

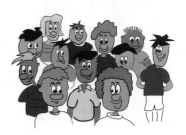

▼
TIP:

Yes. People with diabetes do have special needs for vitamins and minerals. When your blood glucose levels are high, glucose spills into your urine, leading to an increase in urination. This may lead to excessive losses of magnesium, zinc, and water-soluble vitamins such as vitamin C. Also, many people with diabetes are on weight-reduction diets and may not be eating a well-balanced diet. Nonprescription multivitamin and mineral products can be used to replace these possible deficits, but be sure to discuss any additional supplementation with your physician. By eating a well-balanced, healthy diet, many people can obtain their necessary vitamins and minerals and can avoid spending a lot of money on dietary supplements, but others may benefit from their use (see page 96).

I have been reading a lot about antioxidants such as vitamins A, C, and E. Should I be taking these vitamins?

▼
TIP:

It depends. Vitamins A, C, and E are antioxidants that neutralize substances called free radicals that can cause damage to cells throughout the body. Some studies have shown that taking the antioxidant vitamins E and C can protect your heart against heart disease. The recommended dose of vitamin E for heart protection is usually 400 to 800 IU (international units), and the dose of vitamin C is generally 500 to 1,000 mg daily. Since Vitamin E may decrease the ability of your blood to clot, you should not take it if you are also taking a blood thinner such as warfarin (Coumadin). There is less evidence that vitamin A works as well as an antioxidant, and high intakes can build up in the liver and cause toxicity, especially if the dose exceeds 25,000 IU daily. Smokers or former smokers should not take more than the recommended adult daily requirement of Vitamin A (5,000 IU) or excessive beta-carotene (a form of Vitamin A), since this could increase the incidence of lung cancer.

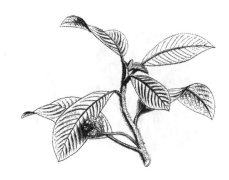

A re *"natural" vitamins more*
effective than synthetic ones?

▼
TIP:

N ot necessarily, but they can be more costly. Synthetic vitamins, or those made by a chemical process, are the exact same molecules as those found in "natural" sources. Your body cannot distinguish between a vitamin derived from a natural or synthetic source. "Natural" or "colloidal" vitamins may be more readily absorbed by your intestines, but vitamin products are standardized to ensure an equivalent amount is absorbed by your gastrointestinal tract. For example, both "natural" and "synthetic" vitamin E contain the same compound. The active compound is measured by international units (IU). Selecting a product based on IU content guarantees that the amount of active ingredient absorbed will be the same, regardless of the vitamin source.

*I've seen chromium advertised a lot by
health food stores. Will it help lower my
blood glucose?*

▼ TIP:

Most likely not. Chromium is a trace mineral that is used by the
body in tiny quantities to regulate glucose metabolism. Most
people have plenty of chromium in their daily meal plans. Some ads
say chromium can lower blood glucose, reduce "sugar cravings,"
reduce weight, and improve insulin sensitivity, but there are few
scientific studies to back up these claims. A chromium deficiency
could lead to elevated blood glucose, but this is extremely rare.
Because chromium deficiency is highly unlikely in most people with
diabetes, routine supplementation is not necessary. If you are
concerned about chromium deficiency, take a multivitamin and
mineral product that contains the recommended daily allowance. If
you choose to take a chromium supplement, make sure your supplement contains only chromium, since some supplements also contain
ingredients that should be avoided by people with diabetes, including ma huang (ephedra) and kola nut (caffeine). Your daily dose of
chromium should not exceed 50 to 200 micrograms.

Chapter 10
COMMON DRUG INTERACTIONS THAT OCCUR WITH MEDICATIONS FOR DIABETES

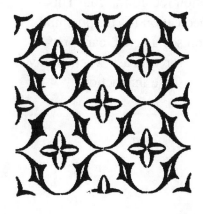

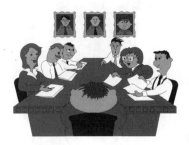

L ately, I have been seen by many physician specialists and each of them has been prescribing medications for me. How will I know if these medications will affect my diabetes or interact with other medications I am taking?

▼
TIP:

This is a difficult problem for many people with diabetes. When reviewing medication profiles, pharmacists commonly identify medications prescribed by various physicians that potentially interact with one another. They also recognize medications that may not be ideal if another medical problem exists. There are several ways for you to help minimize this problem. First, keep your own medication record and show it to every physician and pharmacist you see whenever you are starting a new medication. Second, try to get all of your medications filled at one pharmacy or in a pharmacy network that maintains a single medication record for you. This allows the pharmacist to screen your medication list for potential drug interactions. Finally, every time you see a health care practitioner who prescribes a new medication for you, ask whether any potential exists for a drug-drug or drug-disease interaction.

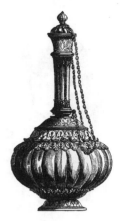

A re there any medications I shouldn't use if I take troglitazone (Rezulin)?

▼
TIP:

Y es. Troglitazone decreases blood levels of oral contraceptives and perhaps estrogen. This could lead to a contraceptive failure resulting in pregnancy or a return of signs of estrogen deficiency, such as hot flashes. If you are taking oral contraceptives, you should stop and use alternative forms of contraception. If this is undesirable, ask your doctor if you should take a different diabetes medication, or if you should take an oral contraceptive with a higher dose of estrogen. Cholestyramine (Questran), a medication used to decrease cholesterol levels, can substantially decrease the amount of troglitazone that is absorbed by the digestive system if you take it at the same time as troglitazone. Troglitazone (Rezulin) is a relatively new medication and because of this, other drug interactions may be discovered as more and more people use it. Therefore, if you are taking troglitazone, ask your pharmacist and physician about potential drug interactions each time a new medication is prescribed for you.

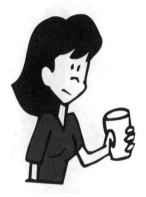

*M*y doctor has just prescribed cisapride
(Propulsid) for my gastroparesis
(diabetic stomach). Is it safe to take this
medication with itraconazole (Sporanox), the
medication I am taking for my toenail
infection?

▼
TIP:

N o. You should not take a combination of these medications
because they can cause dangerous heart rhythms when taken
together. Itraconazole and other medications used to treat fungal
infections decrease the ability of the liver to detoxify medications.
Because of this effect, some medications can accumulate in the body
to dangerous levels. This is the case with cisapride, which can cause
irregular heart rhythms. Alternative medications must be used to
treat your gastroparesis, or you must wait until you have completed
treatment of your toenail infection before you begin taking cisapride. However, you should be aware that it may take several weeks
for your body to eliminate itraconazole completely after you have
stopped taking it.

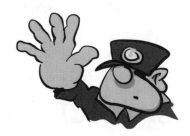

I am on a *"statin" called lovastatin
(Mevacor) to lower my cholesterol.
Are there any medications that I should
avoid?*

▼
TIP:

Yes. There are several prescription medications that can interact
with lovastatin (Mevacor) and other medications that belong to
this group. The other available statins include fluvastatin (Lescol),
pravastatin (Pravachol), simvastatin (Zocor), cerivastatin (Baycol),
and atorvastatin (Lipitor). Your physician and pharmacist will check
the particular statin you are taking for any drug interactions. Gem-
fibrozil (Lopid), a medication that lowers triglyceride levels,
interacts with all of the statins and can lead to a muscle or kidney
disorder on rare occasions. For this reason, many physicians will not
use these two medications together. However, some people with
high levels of cholesterol and triglycerides may take these drugs
together with careful monitoring of their kidney and muscle function. A group of antibiotics used to treat fungal infections
(fluconazole, ketoconazole, and itraconazole) also can cause a
muscle or kidney disorder and should not be given with the statins.
The same is true for the antibiotic erythromycin. The effects of the
blood thinner warfarin (Coumadin) can be enhanced by the statins,
but this can generally be monitored with careful blood testing.

Chapter 11
MISCELLANEOUS INFORMATION

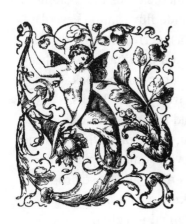

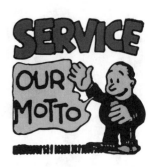

*I receive a bigger discount from my insur-
ance company if I have my prescriptions
filled by mail. What services can I expect?*

▼
TIP:

Many mail-order pharmacies offer good, efficient service when it comes to filling your regular medications. However, most cannot quickly fill prescriptions for medications you need right away, nor are they able to give personalized advice about over-the-counter products. Some have toll-free hot lines to answer your questions about prescriptions they have filled for you or educational programs about diabetes. Ideally, one pharmacy or pharmacy network should have a record of all of the prescription medications you are taking, a history of any bad effects from medications that you have experienced (especially allergies), and your most basic medical history. This allows the pharmacist to screen every new medication that is added to your regimen. Because records of mail-order pharmacies are not always linked to your local pharmacy, potential problems could be missed. You should keep your own detailed medication record (include medication name, strength, dose, and dates of use) and share it with all of your health care providers. Be sure to include nonprescription medications, herbal remedies, vitamins, and minerals in your records.

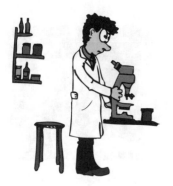

*W*hat qualities should I look for in a pharmacist who oversees my medications?

▼
TIP:

A good pharmacist can be a valuable resource for people with type 2 diabetes because they take more medications than most other people. Therefore, it is important to find a pharmacist who is willing to take the time to review any changes in your medication history each time you get a new prescription and to carefully review the new medication's proper use with you. The pharmacist should also quickly assess whether you are responding to your medications and whether you have developed any common side effects. The pharmacist should advise you about over-the-counter medications in order to avoid side effects or drug-drug interactions. Although many pharmacists are busier than ever, there are still highly qualified pharmacists who are willing to meet with you by appointment to review your medication use and to contact physicians or other health care providers on your behalf. These pharmacists can provide many other services, such as teach you how to use glucose meters, give you immunizations, take your blood pressure, and recommend a product to help you stop smoking.

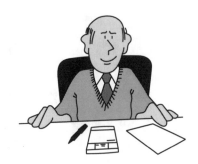

*W*hat questions should I ask my
pharmacist each time I begin
taking a new medication?

▼
TIP:

To protect yourself and to increase the chances that you will get
the best effect from your medications, ask the pharmacist these
questions:

- What is the name of this medication and why am I taking it?
- How should I take it to get the best effect? (For example, with or
  without meals? What time of the day?)
- What good effects can I expect and when?
- How will I know if the medication is working?
- What are the common side effects and how will I know if I have
  them?
- Are there any ways to avoid or diminish these side effects?
- Are there any side effects serious enough to discontinue the
  medication?
- Will my medical conditions make me more susceptible to any of
  this medication's side effects?
- Will this medication interact with any other medications I am
  taking? What is the effect of the interaction?

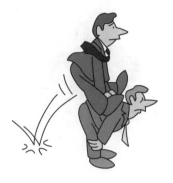

I have been taking Micronase for many years. When I last refilled my prescription, I noticed that the pill was a different color. The pharmacist told me he had filled my prescription with a generic brand because this was covered by my insurance. Is this medication likely to have the same effect as Micronase?

▼
TIP:

Yes. A generic brand of a medication has the same chemical structure as the brand name medication and is provided in the same strength and dosage form (for example, tablet, syrup, or ointment). The Food and Drug Administration has strict standards for manufacturers of generic medications to ensure that they will have the same effects as the brand name medication. Once a medication has lost its patent status, other manufacturers may produce a generic product, and in some cases, the primary source of the generic products is the original manufacturer. Because generic medications are generally less expensive than their brand name equivalents, insurance companies give patients, doctors, and pharmacies incentives to prescribe and dispense generic drugs.

I have been taking lovastatin (Mevacor), but when I refilled my prescription, the pharmacist told me this medication was no longer included in the "formulary" used by my insurance company. I received simvastatin (Zocor), which the pharmacist said worked in the same way. Will this medication have the same effect?

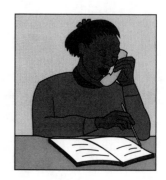

▼
TIP:

You have experienced what the industry calls a "therapeutic interchange." Often, several manufacturers make medications that belong to the same class of agents, have a similar chemical structure, work by the same mechanism, and generally have the same effects. A group of health professional experts pronounces the medications in this group "therapeutically equivalent." The insurance company or HMO then decides which medication to include in the formulary (medications approved for use within a health care insurance plan) based on price. Other factors, such as ease of use (a single daily dose versus a twice daily dose), may also be considered. However, each medication is likely to have a unique dose and dose regimen, and side effects may differ slightly. You should carefully review how to take the medication with your pharmacist and check with your doctor to make sure you are still getting good effects from the new drug.

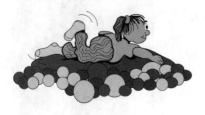

I have several young grandchildren who visit me on occasion. I have asked my pharmacist not to use childproof caps because I have such a hard time opening them. Is there any danger to the children if they accidentally take the medications I use to treat my type 2 diabetes?

▼
TIP:

Yes, depending on the type of medication you are taking. The sulfonylurea medications and repaglinide (Prandin) are most likely to cause acute problems if a child ingests a large amount. These drugs are likely to cause severe hypoglycemia that could last up to 24 hours. High doses of metformin could cause lactic acidosis. Troglitazone (Rezulin) is not likely to cause any acute effects. Acarbose (Precose) may cause temporary abdominal pain, gas, and diarrhea. Nevertheless, whenever an ingestion of any sort is suspected, you should call the local poison control center or the emergency number (911) for advice. Since it is difficult to predict the toxic potential of medications, especially if several medications are taken at once, prevention is key. Take time to store all medications and toxic cleaners out of the reach of children, preferably in a locked cabinet, when you are expecting a visit.

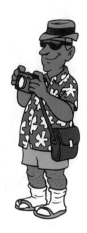

I will be traveling abroad for 4 weeks. What precautions should I take in case I misplace my medications?

▼
TIP:

First, be aware that the medication you are taking may or may not be available in the country to which you are traveling. There is a good chance that even if the medication is available, it will have a different name or will be available in different strengths. Before you leave, you should ask your doctor to provide a letter that briefly describes your medical conditions and their current treatments. Bring extra prescriptions for the medications you are taking so pharmacists or physicians in other countries can provide them for you in an emergency. Write down a detailed list of all the medications you are taking and ask your pharmacist to provide extra supplies of them that you can store in separate bags. Always keep a 2-week supply of medications with you at all times in case your luggage is lost. Make an effort to store all medications in an airtight, insulated case to minimize exposure to temperature and humidity extremes. Finally, wear an ID bracelet and carry an ID in your wallet that identifies you as someone with diabetes.

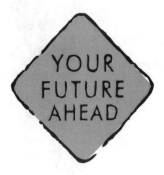

Many members of my family have diabetes, and now I am worried about my children. Are there any medications they can take to prevent or delay the onset of type 2 diabetes?

▼
TIP:

Perhaps. The National Institutes of Health is sponsoring a study called the Diabetes Prevention Program to answer this question. People in the study will be those at high risk for developing diabetes. These individuals have "impaired glucose tolerance." That is, they have blood glucose levels that are higher than normal, but not high enough to be diagnosed with diabetes. People in the study will be assigned to one of three groups for 3 to 6 years. One group will receive a placebo (inactive pill), another group will participate in a diet and exercise program, and the last group will receive metformin (Glucophage). The purpose of the study is to determine if people taking metformin or those assigned to a diet and exercise group are less likely to develop type 2 diabetes over time compared to the group taking a placebo.

GLOSSARY OF TERMS

Acarbose. Precose is the brand name. A member of the alpha-glucosidase inhibitor class of drugs.

Acetohexamide. Dymelor is the brand name. A member of the sulfonylurea class of drugs. Various generic brands are also available.

Alpha-glucosidase Inhibitors. A class of drugs that improves glucose levels after meals by slowing the breakdown of starches to simple sugars that are absorbed by the intestines. Acarbose (Precose) and miglitol (Glyset) are members of this class.

Beta-blockers. Medications often prescribed for people with diabetes who have experienced a heart attack to provide protection against a second attack. These medications are also used to treat high blood pressure, angina (chest pain), glaucoma, and migraine headaches.

Biguanides (bye.gwa.nighds). A class of drugs that improves glucose control by decreasing the production of glucose by the liver. They may also enhance the ability of cells to use glucose. Metformin (Glucophage) is the only member of this class available in the United States.

Brand. A brand name formulation of a medication is the trade name given to a medication by a pharmaceutical company. In order to regain their financial investment in the development and research of a new medication, pharmaceutical companies are given patents for their medications for an average of 7 years following the FDA approval for the medication. This prevents other companies from making generic versions of the same medication until the original patent expires.

Chlorpropamide. Diabinese is the brand name. A member of the sulfonylurea class of drugs. Various generic brands are also available.

DiaBeta. A brand name for glyburide, a member of the sulfonylurea class of drugs.

Diabinese. A brand name for chlorpropamide, a member of the sulfonylurea class of drugs.

Dymelor. A brand name for acetohexamide, a member of the sulfonylurea class of drugs.

Generic. The scientific name for a drug. Generic formulations contain the same chemical as brand name formulations and have equivalent effects.

Glipizide. Glucotrol and Glucotrol XL are brand names of this medication. A member of the sulfonylurea class of drugs.

Glucophage. The brand name for metformin, a member of the biguanide class of drugs.

Glucotrol. A brand name for glipizide, a member of the sulfonylurea class of drugs.

Glyburide. DiaBeta, Glynase, and Micronase are brand names. A member of the sulfonylurea class of drugs. Various generic brands are also available.

Glynase. A brand name for glyburide, a member of the sulfonylurea class of drugs.

Glyset. A brand name for miglitol. A member of the alpha-glucosidase inhibitor class of drugs.

Hyperglycemia. High levels of glucose in the bloodstream. Normal values are between 70 and 140 milligrams/deciliter (mg/dl).

Hypoglycemia. Low levels of glucose in the bloodstream, typically less than 60 milligrams per deciliter (mg/dl). Can be caused by excessive doses of insulin and certain diabetes medications, especially when meals are missed.

Insulin Resistance. An inability to respond to normal levels of insulin. It is associated with obesity, high blood glucose concentrations, high blood pressure, and type 2 diabetes.

Lactic Acidosis. A very rare but serious side effect of metformin that occurs when lactic acid builds up in the bloodstream. People at risk have heart failure or lung, kidney, or liver problems. Symptoms include fast and shallow breathing, muscle pain, and unusual tiredness or weakness.

Meglitinides. A new class of drugs that stimulates the release of insulin from the pancreas, similar to how sulfonylureas work. However, these medications act more quickly and their action is shorter. Currently, repaglinide (Prandin) is the only member of this class of drugs.

Metformin. Glucophage is the brand name. A member of the biguanide class of drugs.

Micronase. A brand name for glyburide, a member of the sulfonylurea class of drugs.

Miglitol. Glyset is the brand name. A member of the alpha-glucosidase inhibitor class of drugs.

Orinase. A brand name for tolbutamide, a member of the sulfonylurea class of drugs.

Prandin. A brand name for repaglinide, a member of the meglitinide class of drugs.

Precose. A brand name for acarbose, a member of the alpha-glucosidase inhibitor class of drugs.

Repaglinide. Prandin is the brand name. A member of a new class of drugs, the meglitinides.

Rezulin. The brand name for troglitazone, a member of the thiazolidinedione class of drugs.

Sulfonylureas (sole.fa.nil.your.ee.uz). A class of drugs that decreases blood glucose by increasing insulin release from the pancreas. Medications in this class include acetohexamide, chlorpropamide, glimepiride, glipizide, glyburide, tolbutamide, and tolazamide.

Statins. A term used to describe a class of drugs that decreases blood cholesterol and triglyceride levels. They also increase levels of the good (HDL) cholesterol. Examples of medications in this class include lovastatin (Mevacor), pravastatin (Pravachol), and simvastatin (Zocor).

Thiazolidinediones (thigh.uh.zole.eh.deen.dye.owns). A class of drugs that improves glucose control by enhancing the action of insulin. Consequently, the body is able to use glucose more efficiently. Currently, troglitazone (Rezulin) is the only member of this class. Other medications in this class are likely to be introduced.

Tolbutamide. Orinase is the brand name. A member of the sulfonylurea class of drugs. Various generic brands are also available

Tolinase. A brand name for tolazamide, a member of the sulfonylurea class of drugs.

Troglitazone. Rezulin is the brand name. A member of a new class of drugs, the thiazolidinediones.

INDEX

Humulin, 55
Hydrochlorothiazide, patients taking, 82
Hypoglycemia, 28
  monitoring symptoms of, 27, 33, 64, 81
  reducing risk of, 44, 51–52
  treating, 34
  while taking repaglinide, 39

I
ID bracelet, 111
Impotence, treating, 72
Injections
  lumps from, 65
  overcoming fear of, 11, 43
  preparing ahead, 60
  sites for, 59, 65
Insulin. *See also* individual types of insulin
  high doses of, 51
  mixing types of, 45, 48, 60
  storing, 54, 60–61
  types of, 44–48
Insulin analog, 47
Insulin pumps, 49
Insulin therapy, 2, 5, 44
  adjusting with exercise, 56
  avoiding, 11
  delaying, 43
  initiating, 41
  innovations in, 57
  in pregnancy, 22
  side effects of, 62–65
  timing, 44–46, 49, 64
  in type 2 diabetes, 40–57
  while breastfeeding, 22
Itraconazole, cautions for patients taking cisapride, 102

K
Kidney function, and diabetes, 23, 69, 74
Kidney X-rays, for patients taking metformin, 37

L
Lactic acidosis, 23–24, 36
Lanoxin, patients taking, 24

Lasix, patients taking, 24
Lente insulin, 44, 55, 60, 64
Lispro insulin, 45–48, 54–55
Liver function, 32, 35, 87
Lovastatin, cautions for patients taking, 103

M
Medication, non-prescription, warnings with, 84–98
Medication record, maintaining, 100, 111
Medications for treating diabetes. *See also* Insulin therapy; individual medications
  action of, 4, 76–83
  adjusting during holiday eating, 16
  adjusting with exercise, 20
  availability while traveling, 111
  "best," 7
  during breastfeeding, 22
  changing, 41–42, 106, 109
  combining, 10, 12, 42
  cost of, 7, 105, 108
  cross-reactivity of, 25
  different actions of, 2
  half-life of, 26
  interactions of, 21, 75, 99–103
  minimizing dose of, 9
  missing a dose, 15
  names of, 3
  oral, 5, 27
  potency of, 6
  during pregnancy, 22
  protecting children from, 110
  side effects of, 7, 12, 29–39, 106–107
  storing, 54, 60–61, 111
  taking with food, 17
  treating complications of diabetes, 66–75
  when to take, 19, 26
  and X ray tests, 37
Menstrual periods resuming, while taking troglitazone, 32
Metformin, 3–4, 6–7, 13, 51
  and congestive heart failure, 24
  and kidney function, 23, 36
  and kidney X rays, 37
  side effects of, 38

taking, 17, 19, 27–28
taking maximum dose of, 43
Mevacor, cautions for patients taking, 103
Microalbuminuria, 69
Micronase, 3, 108
Miglitol, 3–4, 6–7
  missing a dose of, 15
  taking, 17, 19
Multivitamins, patients taking, 83

N
Names of medications, 3. *See also*
  individual medications
Nasal congestion, treating, 89
National Institutes of Health, Diabetes
  Prevention Program of, 112
Nausea, 70
  while taking troglitazone, 32
Nervousness. *See* Hypoglycemia
Niacin, and diabetes, 77, 83
Nonprescription medications, 84–98,
  106
  sugar content of, 90
  warnings labels on, 85, 92
Nonsteroidal anti-inflammatory agents
  (NSAIDS), and diabetes, 92
NPH insulin, 44–45, 48, 55, 60, 64

O
Obesity, 51, 75
Oral medications, 5, 51
  switching to, 53
Orinase, 3
Over-the-counter medications, 84–98,
  106

P
Peripheral vascular disease, cautions for
  patients with, 79
Pharmacist, consulting with, 71, 86–87,
  92, 100–101, 103, 105–110
Phenylpropanolamine, cautions
  concerning, 94
Polycystic ovary disease, patients with,
  32
Postmenopausal patients, 80
Potency of medications, 6
Prandin, 3, 7
  missing a dose of, 15

missing a meal with, 28
side effects of, 39
taking, 17, 19
toxic potential of, 110
Precose, 3, 7
  missing a dose of, 15
  taking, 17, 19
Pregnancy, and diabetes, 22
Premixed insulin, 48
Propulsid, cautions for patients taking
  itraconazole, 102
Protease inhibitors, and diabetes, 77

R
Rapid-acting insulin, 45–48
Red pepper cream, 68
Regular insulin, 45–48, 54–55
Repaglinide, 3–4, 6–7
  missing a dose of, 15
  missing a meal with, 28
  side effects of, 39
  taking, 17, 19
  toxic potential of, 110
Rezulin, 3, 51–52
  cautions for patients taking, 101
  side effects of, 32, 35
  taking, 17

S
Sexual side effects, treating, 72
Shakiness. *See* Hypoglycemia
Side effects of medications, 7, 12,
  29–39, 106–107
Site of action of medications, 4
Sites for injections, 59, 65
Skin, yellowing of. *See* Liver function
Smoking, and diabetes, 96
Sore throat. *See* Liver function
Sporanox, cautions for patients taking
  cisapride, 102
Statins, cautions for patients taking,
  103
Stomach pain, 70
  while taking acarbose, 30
  while taking metformin, 38
Strength of medications, 6
Sulfa antibiotics, patients allergic to, 25
Sweating. *See* Hypoglycemia
Syndrome X, 75